THE LONG ROAD CALLED GOODBYE

THE LONG ROAD CALLED GOODBYE

TRACING THE COURSE OF ALZHEIMER'S

by

CHARLOTTE AKIN

CREIGHTON UNIVERSITY PRESS
Omaha, Nebraska
Association of Jesuit University Presses

Library of Congress Cataloging in Publication Data

Akin, Charlotte, 1948-
    The long road called goodbye : tracing the course of
    Alzheimer's / by Charlotte Akin.
        p. cm.
    Includes bibliographical references.
    ISBN 1-881871-33-9 (hc) -- ISBN 1-881871-34-7 (pbk.)
    1. Alzheimer's disease--Case studies. 2. Alzheimer's
    disease--Patients--Care. I. Title

    RC523.2 .A43 2000
    362.1'96831--dc21
                                                    00-025772

EDITORIAL   MARKETING & DISTRIBUTION
Creighton University Press   Fordham University Press
2500 California Plaza   University Box L
Omaha, Nebraska 68178   Bronx, New York 10458

Printed in the United States of America

For Ralph, my closest traveling companion.
He went the whole distance.

Contents

Acknowledgments

We were driving on a two-lane stretch of I-90, my young husband and I, in the hilly rangeland between Vantage and Ellensburg, Washington. Both of us had worked all week, and it was nearly midnight on a Friday night. We were going to visit friends and family in Seattle. There was a blizzard raging on this dark night; the going was slow. As we came around a bend in the road, there was a deserted car on the shoulder. Just as we passed it, I said, "Ralph, I think I saw movement in that car!" Without a word, Ralph pulled our car off the road and proceeded very carefully to back up onto the shoulder, around another corner, until we got near the other car. It was a treacherous move. Suddenly there was a man, nearly hysterical, telling us that he, his wife, and their infant had been freezing for hours with not so much as a taillight working in their car. They had given up hope that anyone would stop. Of course they bundled in with us. I stayed with the woman and child when we got to Ellensburg, until Ralph made sure a tow had been sent and that the man had what he needed for his family for the night.

The road that is Alzheimer's Disease is likewise a treacherous road. There is danger to financial well-being, to relationships, and to care-giver health. Surviving the care of my mother—without guilt, without bitterness, without the ruination of my own health—was no small feat. It could not have been done without help from others. Consistent help, determined help, conscious help, freely given. I came to depend upon this; I had no other choice. My husband of over thirty years now, Ralph never varied in his willingness to assist me or my parents. Though he would say it is nothing more than just the right way to live, his countless acts of kindness and his unselfish spirit were an inspiration to me.

The act of juggling children at home, a full-time career, responsibility for the care of Mother, management of a home, and attention to my husband was an enormous task. While I had a housekeeper a few hours a week, my children, The Incredible Akin Sisters, could be counted on to fill in, help out, and do additional chores. I could count on Heather (now Heather McConley) to comfort me and Janelle to humor me. They both took turns at endless errands. Most of all, they helped by being good people. They saved me the worry that many parents have.

In addition, my family listened when I needed to talk. Sometimes when I was upset or trying to work through a thorny ethical issue, this must have seemed tedious and morose. They would listen to me talk it through, and then they would have to listen again as I called long-distance to talk it over with other friends or relatives. They never told me that they were sick of hearing about Mother, although there were times when they surely were. Ralph, especially, was an amazing sounding board. I could trust his clear thinking, his strong integrity.

Finally, my family had to share me. There were times I could not visit my daughter, Heather, at school at Willamette University because I was sick, exhausted, or overwhelmed. Janelle, my youngest, gave up time with me that can never be recovered.

I am deeply grateful for the generosity of spirit and the helping hands that were part of my daily life with Ralph, Janelle, and Heather. Only a fraction of their support and astonishing honesty is chronicled here.

One of the things that is sometimes needed is for people to just get out of the way. Despite every good intention, there are times when people can't or won't help. At these times, it is most helpful if they just step aside. Alzheimer's is not a disease that everyone can handle being around. Janelle had a hard time being around Mother, for example. Ralph did, too, at the end especially. I feel fortunate that some of my relatives had the grace at these times to just let me take care of things.

Many colleagues and friends told me of families who were counterproductive during tough times. Not only did they not help, they hurt. They complained, felt that they could be doing so much better, and let everyone know it. I *never* experienced this. My extended family was positive and constructive. My brothers, John and Tom Leonard, gave me carte-blanche in taking care of Mother. They spoke highly and gratefully of me. They gave me solid support, start to finish. John took care of all of my mother's finances after our father passed away. Tom attended to the estate sale, the cleaning, and re-carpeting of their home. His family also provided great vacation times for Ralph and me.

Because this book is a case study wrapped in a story, the purpose of this book is to educate, not just to entertain or remember. Given this purpose, the necessity for honesty—sometimes in intensely personal areas—is greater. My whole family—husband, children, brothers, and sister, Mary Lou Stowell—had to be willing to expose some of themselves. As I anguished over who and what to reveal, how much to expose, I was sustained by one thought. My mother herself would have censored none of it. She would have laid herself bare to make a contribution to the knowledge of this disease. I and all who read and learn from this book are indebted to those who shared themselves in this way. Some of the names of the residents of caregiving facilities and their relatives have been changed to protect their privacy.

My two aunts, Aunt Babe (Gudrun Layton) and Auntie Ethel (Ethel Van Dyke) were also sources of comfort and help. I struggled with whether or not I should quit my job and take Mother into my home. My Auntie Ethel could tell me what she knew Mom had wanted. When Heather got married, I agonized over whether to bring Mother to the wedding. Aunt Babe could advise me on how Mother would prefer to be treated. Both aunts helped me think through the ethical issues that arose.

Unfailing help came also from a number of friends. I don't know what I would have done without Mom and Dad's best friends, Homer and Betty Schmitt. I sought their wise counsel often, and they were so thoughtful and gracious. Although they lived in Seattle, three hours to the north, they visited Mom often enough to give me feedback on her care and progress. So close to a situation that was intense and consuming, I sometimes needed the advice of those who loved her, but who stood back just a little from it.

I deeply appreciate the help I got from a number of professionals. Connie Easter was the administrator of the Cascade Inn, a retirement community. Professionals at the University of Washington, where my mother was part of a long-term study, included Meredith Pfanschmidt, the nurse in charge of the Alzheimer's study, and Zilpha Haycox, Lead Psychometrist. Dr. Richard Moller, our family dentist, patiently guided us through a series of procedures and months of work to restore Mother's mouth after years of neglect. Dr. Manuella Laderas, Mother's internist, broke all the molds. An exceptional listener, she went so far as to give me her home phone number. She visited Mom in her foster care home. Dr. Laderas went out of her way to be there for us as an excellent physician who walked with us to the end.

Special thanks also go to my editor, Brent Spencer, first for appreciating this book, and then for helping to make it better. He added greatly to the quality of the work.

Thanks also to my good friend, Dr. Sharon Hartnett. Sharon was working on her doctorate as I was working on this book. We encouraged, helped, and believed in each other. Thanks also to Howard Gruetzner for the help I found in his book and for his support of mine.

Finally, I am eternally indebted to Annabelle and Ken Rhodes. Ann managed an adult foster care home in her own home, and Ken graciously put up with it! Ann took such loving care of Mom; I could not have made it through this without her. She was helped by Ana Bordea, a recent Romanian immigrant, who knows how to love, nurture, and tend—gifts that transcend language and culture. Janice Ripp also worked at Annabelle's Foster Care Home during Mother's last year. Janice brought intelligence, capability, and spiritual support to her work. For the loving, warm, fun, and secure atmosphere these people provided my mother, there are no words. When I think of them still, they give me hope.

Charlotte A. Akin
Battle Ground, WA

Introduction

When I was five years old, in 1953, my mother took me to South Dakota to visit my aunt and grandmother. I have only one memory of the trip. My Aunt Dagny took me to school with her for a day. She was a teacher in a one-room school house. She taught eight grades and stoked the wood stove. Watching her teach and being in that classroom felt to me like *home*. I knew forever after that I was born to teach.

Of course I became a teacher. I've taught preschoolers to adults. So I am always bothered when I come upon information that people truly need that is in a format they are unlikely to access, such as medical journals. I wonder, *How could I teach this and make it interesting?*

When my mother was diagnosed with Alzheimer's Disease, I wanted to learn three things. First, I wanted to know the course of the disease. How long does this last? What will happen to my mother over time? These questions are important not just to satisfy curiosity. The answers affect legal and financial decisions. They give some idea of the care that will be needed in the future.

The second question was, "How does this disease impact family members?" How do people cope with seeing a loved one degenerate ever so slowly? Are there any strategies that might help with this? How do children react to the disease? How do family members respond to one another when some react to illness by withdrawing? Could my ailing father take care of a wife with Alzheimer's? How much and what kind of help would be needed from other family members? There are many layers to the impact of Alzheimer's upon a family.

Third, I wanted to find out what good care looked like. I wanted to know the options. Would in-home care be best? An institution? Should I move Mother in with me? What costs are involved? Does care even matter to the person with Alzheimer's? What *would* matter to my mother?

These were the questions I tried to answer by reading medical books, caregiver books, memoirs, and by living with this disease. Once I found answers, there remained the question: *How could I teach the information to others and make it interesting for them?* What kind of format would people be most comfortable reading? The answer: I could do a full-term, start-to-finish case study and write it as a *story.*

Any medical disease or psycho-social disorder generally has a cluster of symptoms. Each afflicted individual manifests most, but not all, of those symptoms. So while a case study would not necessarily cover every single thing that might happen, it covers many things—and those in depth.

A case study is a way of illuminating clinical information by making it personal and giving it a setting. It looks at one person's experience in depth over time. Through the power of story, the reader is taken on a journey that chronicles the disease. Occasionally in this story I want to highlight one aspect of Alzheimer's by showing several examples over the course of a year. Then, as the story resumes, it goes back to an earlier date. While the time line may be briefly interrupted, this gives the reader a closer look at some critical issues.

I was tempted to begin the story at the beginning of Alzheimer's Disease, or even later, when caregiving became an issue that impacted the family. But there was the realization that so much of what helped me to help my mother was knowing *her* history. Alzheimer's robs a person first of recent memories, then gradually of more distant ones. Knowing about Mother's early life on a farm, for example, gave me the idea of taking her into the country for drives when she was "way far back" with the disease. Her eyes yearned, then, to see fields and barns. Instead of taking her to a grocery store to buy apples, I drove her a few extra miles to a farm's produce stand. We sang old songs. So Mother's story is best told with a brief description of her beginnings to give the reader a sense of the woman who was—before there was Alzheimer's Disease.

I was also tempted to write this story without much family history. After all, nobody needs to know the family's business—the good, the bad, and the ugly. There were two important reasons to include the context of family, however. First, family is an Alzheimer's victim's primary human resource, as he or she increasingly has less ability to function. Second, people coping with Alzheimer's need hope. I did not want readers to feel that while *our* family somehow struggled through this, theirs would not be able to. No family is perfect, and Alzheimer's does not wait for the perfect time and place to strike. So without necessarily divulging all the family secrets, I did include enough of a sketch to give a realistic picture of how one family, however flawed, made their way along the road.

The road, of course, is Alzheimer's Disease. Its length is measured in years. Some sources break this illness into three clinical stages. The amnestic stage primarily describes early memory loss. The dementia stage is the middle stage that deals with cognitive (learning, reasoning) problems and emotional upheaval. The final vegetative stage is where the patient is unable to care for himself entirely. For instructional reasons, I chose a source which breaks this long road into five stages.

There are people on the road. The traveler is a victim of Alzheimer's Disease. The cadre of caregivers—family, friends, and professionals—is the vehicle that supports and helps the traveler as the long journey progresses.

The Early Confusional Stage

The first stage of Alzheimer's is difficult to detect. The victim may just be a little forgetful. Recent events and conversations are most affected. These are the things that happened earlier in the day, yesterday, perhaps last week. The person may unconsciously repeat himself or herself, though usually is able to compensate and cover up a gradually worsening memory.

Driving reactions may be slightly slower. Driving to familiar locations is not a problem. Traveling to a new place is. A person may easily become lost in unfamiliar territory.

The person may have less initiative socially. He or she may be less tactful and/or spontaneous in social situations, often using denial as a coping mechanism, which causes others to underestimate the severity of symptoms. There may be widely separated events of irrational behavior. Emotionally, the person may seem slightly unhappy or anxious, but others are mystified, since the causes for these emotional changes are not clear.

The kinds of problems that appear in this first stage of Alzheimer's Disease are subtle. They can be easily dismissed, laughed off, hidden, and denied. Alzheimer's is not usually diagnosed at this early stage (Gruetzner, 1984).

This is a summary of the clinical definition of the first stage of Alzheimer's in Howard Gruetzner's book, *Alzheimer's: A Caregiver's Guide and Sourcebook*. The coming chapters will illustrate how this *looked* and how it played out in my mother's life. Dates are included as mile-markers, to give a sense of time, to measure the length of the road. This format will be repeated throughout the journey.

Chapter 1

Family

Unlike other trips I've taken, the journey with Alzheimer's had a shadowy beginning. It's hard to pinpoint the date that I joined my mother on this road, hard to say when she began it. Certainly it began before I started gathering information, before I was confronted with all the problems of providing care for her. In a way, it even began before I went to visit my Aunt Dagny.

"Do you think your mother is happy?" she had asked, suddenly quite serious.

We were sitting in a cozy mobile home in Idaho Falls, Idaho. She was recovering from cancer surgery, and I had traveled here to see her. Her place was nothing special, just a neatly kept single-wide in a mobile home park where she lived with her husband, Jim. She had taught school for forty-three years and raised seven children. And she could tell a tale like nobody else. So we sat there together in the living room darkened by wood paneling, and she sat back and talked for the better part of three days. I could have listened to my Aunt Dagny for months, learning the lessons woven between the lines.

All five of the Anderson children had been born in a one-room sod house on the prairie of South Dakota, the children of homesteaders, immigrants from Norway. Their mother, short and plump, actually gave birth to six children. One of them, Agnes, had died of appendicitis at the age of four, so my mother, who came later, was also named Agnes in order to honor her paternal grandmother. Their tall and dark-haired father, John Anderson, was a stern and serious man. He helped build the Lutheran church near the tiny town of Lemmon, cared for his neighbors, and was involved in local politics. After befriending a man who died leaving no family, the struggling immigrants inherited a home. They gratefully moved into larger quarters. By then "Little Agnes" was five.

Life was simple. Little Agnes had few playmates and fewer toys—a prized shoe box and a doll, Pethernella, which she shared with her cousin, Magnihild, who lived on a neighboring farm. Out on the stark and endless prairie, she played "funeral" with her two brothers and sisters, Dagny and Gudrun—called "Babe" for the obvious reason. Her older brother, Einar, tall and brooding like his father, was always the minister. Little Agnes played a mourner, because she could cry. The actors changed roles from time to time. Often Babe was the deceased, and Dagny and another brother, Arne, might be the mourning parents. Without television or many books, this was the kind of drama familiar to the isolated farm children growing up.

With children from neighboring farms, they learned to smoke and kiss behind the barn. They learned to drive a Model A on a frozen river bed, making Little Agnes a nervous driver for life. Their father played the fiddle. Neighbors sometimes gathered for a dance, to sing, or tell stories. It was no surprise, then, that Dagny became a marvelous story teller, Babe was known for her beautiful singing voice, and Little Agnes never lost her love for a dance.

When their brothers finished eighth grade, they went to work on the farm, and there they spent the rest of their lives. When Dagny finished eighth grade she went on to high school. Their mother was mystified at why a girl would want an education, but Agnes followed suit, moving to a nearby town and living with a family as their maid until she could graduate. A neighbor loaned Dagny money for college. When she finished, she gave Agnes money for college. When Agnes finished, she gave money to Babe. Babe paid back the neighbor. All three became teachers in one-room schoolhouses in South Dakota. All three later moved beyond the borders of their home state.

Agnes worked as a teacher for six years, and Babe also taught off and on for several years, living all over the world with a husband in the military. Dagny alone made teaching her lifelong profession.

Dagny talked and fixed lunch for us. She wouldn't let me cook; even in poor health, she was the boss of her own kitchen. She and Jim would in poor health, she was the boss of her own kitchen. She and Jim would have a little nap after lunch, while I would go for a walk. Afterwards, she would tell me the stories of the children she taught, throwing back her head for a good laugh from time to time. One had told her she was beautiful. Dagny never put much stock in her looks; this expression of love from a child amused her.

As the days and stories began to wind down, Aunt Dagny asked me, "Do you think your mother is happy?" At the time I knew *some* of where the question was coming from. My parents lived in a large and beautiful brick home overlooking Puget Sound in the suburbs south of Seattle. Cool breezes scented with the salt water wafted through open windows in summers. In winter, fog and drizzle from the water blanketed the neighborhood, and tall evergreens tempered the wind. Even then there was a softness in the atmosphere that surrounded them when compared to the harsh winters and hot summers of Idaho. My parents, while not truly wealthy, were very comfortable in their retirement. They traveled widely and had many friends. Mother was habitually cheerful and also enjoyed perfect health. She was into health and exercise long before it was popular. In the morning at her house, if she wasn't on a brisk walk to the beach, she was exercising with music on the radio or TV. Yet here was her ailing sister asking me if I thought she was happy.

What I *didn't* know at this time was that my Aunt Babe had been openly insulted by my mother a couple of times in the past few years. Babe had told Dagny about it. I also didn't know about an incident that happened at a family reunion in 1982. It included friends from South Dakota as well as relatives. The first day of the reunion was hosted in a spacious home overlooking Lake Coeur d'Alene in Northern Idaho. It was a lovely summer day, so people gathered on the deck outside as well as in the living areas of the house. Both Aunt Dagny and Aunt Babe were there with their husbands. My cousin Pee Wee was there with her twin sister, Fatty. Of course these are not their real names. Daughters of Aunt Dagny, one twin was thin, the other plump at birth. My mother had nicknamed them then and there, and the nicknames stuck. Their names are Marlene and Maxine. Maxine, who is Pee Wee to me, is quite tall. Marlene, who will always be Fatty to me, is not at all fat. But both of them are lots of fun at a party, regardless of what they're called. At the reunion Mother saw Fatty and gave her a big hug. She looked right at Pee Wee without the slightest hint of recognition in her eyes. Pee Wee was quite hurt. It took *over two hour*s before Mother looked at Pee Wee as though she had just come, recognized her, and gave her a big hug.

This incident was important from a couple of perspectives. First, it was not just a moment of forgetfulness, common to all of us. It lasted quite some time, and it occurred with someone Mother knew well and loved. Pee Wee had once lived with our family. Furthermore, when Pee Wee later tried to tell her own mother that Mom didn't recognize her, Aunt Dagny got mad at Pee Wee for saying such a thing! Pee Wee was hurt again. We came to understand much later that this was actually a common reaction of people when told about Mother having Alzheimer's. It was at first hard for people to believe. There is a stigma and a horror to losing one's mind. Friends and family alike would react in a kind of angry denial, mad at the messenger.

But now, a few years later, Dagny herself was sensing that *some*thing was wrong with her sister. Although she was battling cancer in her humble home, it was clear that Dagny was at peace. She was happy. Was her sister? And why was I, all of a sudden, being asked to evaluate my mother? Lately my dad had been asking a different question: "How do you think your mother looks? Do you think she has lost weight?" He'd asked that of me several times in the past few months. Each time I'd told him that I thought she looked great. No, she didn't look thin.

Well, compared to Dad, of course she *was* thin. An epic figure, he was larger than life in many ways. Always playful and the life of any party, he was a huge man, over six feet tall and weighing more than 300 pounds. Mom was forever trying to get him to lose weight. She was an avid reader and a particular interest was nutrition. It dovetailed nicely with her bent for exercise. So she read, dieted, exercised, and preached a bit, too. And Dad dutifully, gratefully ate whatever his fit wife fixed for him before leaving for the office each day. What he didn't say was that "the office" he was referring to was a nearby Winchell's Doughnut shop. He never seemed to mind Mother's preaching and special diets for him, as long as they didn't seriously interfere with his eating.

Dad had met my mother through his best friend, Homer. Dad and Homer grew up in Kansas during the Depression. Charles "Bud" Leonard was as tall as Homer was short, as rough around the edges as Homer was smooth. Bud's father had been the town drunk and had run off with a woman, leaving Bud and his brother, sisters, and mother to fend for themselves. Still, Bud was eternally optimistic, athletic, bright, and more entertaining company than anyone else around. Bud's oldest sister, Lilian, moved to Seattle and married. Bud visited her once, and when he returned to Kansas, he went straight to Homer, pulled him off a tractor, and told him the streets of Seattle were paved in gold. Homer left Kansas and moved to Seattle with Bud.

Soon Homer had a girlfriend named Betty. She was living with her sister and another young woman named Agnes, whom they had met at a bookkeeping school in Wenatchee, a small Central Washington town. Agnes had been a teacher but decided to move West and do office work. Together the three young women went to Seattle to find work. It was only a matter of time before Homer and Betty introduced their roommates to one another. Agnes was not impressed with Bud, the young man who slapped her on the knee during a funny part in the movie. But somehow his rough, boyish charm eventually captivated her, because in 1942 she married him.

Bud and Agnes had their first child just before Bud went to France in World War II. Agnes took her baby, Mary Lou, to South Dakota for a time and lived with her parents. Then she went back to Seattle and settled in with Bud's sister, Lilian, who was also raising a young daughter while her husband was overseas. After the War, Bud settled his growing family in Seattle. Four children grew up in our family. After Mary Lou, I was born second. Then came John, named for his maternal grandfather, and finally Tom.

Mom and Dad established their young family in a middle-class neighborhood on Beacon Hill. Dad became a buyer for Sears. Mom stayed at home raising children in a close-knit neighborhood of like-minded families. We spent Thanksgiving with Homer and Betty's family and other holidays with Auntie Lil (Dad's sister Lilian) and her family.

Dad bought a small dairy farm in Ellensburg in the Yakima River Valley, a two-hour drive from Seattle over to the east side of the Cascade

Mountains. Managers lived full-time in the big farmhouse, while our family had a one-room cabin with a wood stove. Mother packed us up for trips to the farm nearly every weekend. Friday nights or early Saturday mornings found the six of us bundled together in the car singing songs with the radio, playing car games, putting on chains mid-trip in the winter, fighting, laughing, and sleeping along the way.

On the farm we had a different life than the one near the center of Seattle. Dad shed business suits and ties for his blue striped bib overalls. Entrepreneurial in spirit, he was the consummate sidewalk supervisor in a boyish, Tom Sawyer sort of way. Working for Bud was a privilege. When the hay needed to be cut on the farm, Dad could get his city slicker buddies from Sears to don overalls and spend weekends cutting hay. Homer, by now also a Seattle businessman, was good natured enough to keep his farming skills sharp in this way, too.

Mother cooked on the wood stove in the country and enjoyed all the modern conveniences in her home in the city. And while we lived in a close, multi-ethnic neighborhood on Beacon Hill, there was no end to the fun we had just as a family on the farm. We learned to ride a horse. Yes, one horse. We took turns. Because Tom and John were younger and small, they learned to ride calves, too. A big rope hung from the ceiling of the old red barn. We stood in the loft and swung from it. Mary Lou and I converted an old chicken coop into a playhouse and outfitted it with apple crate cupboards and old dishes from the Goodwill store. John and Tom could target practice with a BB gun. We all learned to swim in a large irrigation ditch that ran through the property. Eternally modest, I even went skinny-dipping once in the night with Mary Lou and one of her friends when we'd slept outside under the stars. Among my favorite memories is Mother sliding down a snow-covered hill on a bedpan she'd found at Goodwill.

Resourceful to a fault, Mom used the farm as her classroom. If a cow was about to give birth, for example, she would herd her children to the loft of the barn. We would lie down flat on our stomachs and peep over the edge to the cow below. We would have to be ever so quiet while we watched; we were not allowed to disturb the cow. The family grew close taking those trips over the mountains to the farm. Between that and Beacon Hill, it was the best of both worlds.

In addition to these warm memories, there was a shadow over our family. Its name was alcoholism. Like his father, Dad had a drinking problem that wrought havoc in our lives. Sweet as life was on Beacon Hill and the farm, there were times of horror, too: waking up in the morning to see my father sleeping drunk in the street outside our home, having Dad come to our Christmas programs at church falling-down drunk, seeing my mother's tears as she worked at the kitchen window. These were just a few of the potent signals that all was not well in the Leonard home.

In 1960 Dad sold the farm. We also moved to a suburban community on a Puget Sound beach that year. It was the beginning of a very bleak time in the history of our family. Here the neighbors were strangers who hadn't known us all our lives. The following year Dad's sister, Lilian, died of cancer after suffering for many years. Soon after the move, Dad had back surgery and then left Sears for a variety of jobs. He was a manufacturer's rep and insurance manager. Then he bought a "café" in a run-down industrial part of Seattle. Small and dingy, it was the kind of place that served sandwiches at lunch time and a lot of beer. The teenage girls who waited tables were his daughters. A year or two later Dad sold the place and started a wholesale toy business. Mother kept the books, and John and I both worked in the warehouse as stockmen, filling orders, unloading trucks, and moving merchandise. Nevertheless, the business failed, bankrupting the family in 1967, my second year of college. By that time Dad's drinking was so severe that Mother filed for divorce, and they were separated.

But Dad also had an invincible quality. After his back surgery, the doctors told him he'd never walk again. Coached and coaxed by his children, he was walking within a few months. He went bankrupt in mid-life. The bank gave him six months to raise enough money to save our house. We lost everything, but Dad saved the house and found an occupation for himself in real estate that was better for him in every way. When his wife started divorce proceedings against him after twenty-some years of alcoholism, he quit drinking and won her back. People appreciated Dad for his mind and his many social skills. But those who were really close to him respected him most because he just never gave up. He could seem to be down for the count and somehow come up again swinging.

Dad was forever fun and funny. He was mathematically brilliant. When his mathematical mind wasn't being exercised in business, or counting cows, or figuring milk production, it was being expressed at playing cards. Saturday nights he often spent with his friends playing poker or bridge, depending on the group. Totally unpretentious, rough around the edges, he knew a *zillion* people, and *everybody*, high or low, truly loved him. Often when someone called him on the phone and said, "How are you?" he responded with, "Well, I'm lovable." And so he was.

Certainly he was adored by his wife who was his companion in business and life. After the farm was sold, Mom went camping and fishing. She went to New York City, Alaska, and anywhere else Dad seemed to need to go. She also took trips to South Dakota with anyone who would go with her. She went to Norway with a childhood friend. While she loved her home, "Little Agnes" was known as a good sport who was ready and willing to go just about anywhere.

Mother also took her children to church. On Beacon Hill we went to the Congregational Church. After the move to the suburbs, we went to St. Paul's of Shorewood Lutheran Church. Disenchanted with the organized church from childhood, Dad rarely went. But Mother had her children in Sunday School as soon as they could walk, and she was not opposed to taking a carload of neighborhood children along as well.

Undoubtedly rooted in her faith was a basic integrity that, in spite of our differences, I always respected. The wisdom of Alcoholics Anonymous states that girls raised in alcoholic families either marry one or become one. Mary Lou and I never did either. Mother never let us believe that excessive drinking was acceptable. Somehow she balanced that with an enduring love for Dad which we never—not even during divorce proceedings and separation—doubted.

Mom loved to learn, and so she took classes. She took sewing classes, short hand classes, bookkeeping classes, downhill ski lessons (when she was sixty), real estate classes, cooking classes, yoga classes, aerobics, and Bible study classes.

She was also a reader—not a particular reader—just a reader. She knew from her unending reading a little about a lot of things. An expert at home remedies, I'm sure this interest began when she was a girl back in South developed an interest in medical research and nutrition and was aware of alternative medicines decades before any of these became popular.

Mother's perfect health was documented by a medical history consisting of some fillings and bridgework done on her teeth. She'd also had a little bladder repair done vaginally when she was in her fifties, needed because of seven pregnancies. (She'd had two miscarriages and a stillbirth in addition to her four children.) The doctor took out her uterus at the same time, for convenience. The surgery was done on a Tuesday. I arrived at 10:00 P.M. Friday to help, having traveled 300 miles after work from my home in Spokane. Mom was up vacuuming when I got there. In her late fifties or early sixties, she lost her sense of smell. We never knew why. She had an eternally sunny disposition and always said that if she had to lose one of her senses, smell was perhaps the easiest one to lose. And that was it, until she was nearly 70 years old. She very rarely even got colds or the flu.

In our family we all had nicknames. Tom was called Pooh for a while after Mother read *Winnie the Pooh* to the family out loud. John, who had a more serious nature, was Eeyore. But we made up Mom's nickname ourselves. She was The Doctor Agnes, K.E. (Knows Everything). Given all her classes, remedies, and reading habits, it was no wonder.

As Dad was now in a financially comfortable retirement, his battle with alcohol behind him, the question was: Was this wife of his happy? His answer to my Aunt Dagny would have been, "Hell, yes. Except for that business with Mary Lou . . . "

Authorities on children of alcoholics say that predictable patterns and roles develop in these families. Mary Lou's unfortunate role was that of the "child" who acts out problems and rebels, becoming the scapegoat for the real problems facing the family. Dad never got any help for his alcoholism. He just quit drinking. He never understood either the problem or the related family dynamics, though he had lived with them all his life. As a consequence, he never understood Mary Lou.

Mary Lou was born when Dad was on his way to France in World War II. Mother took a train to meet him in Chicago soon after Mary Lou was born, so he could see her. He didn't return until after she was over a year old. Somehow Mom got it into her head that Dad and Mary Lou could not old. Somehow Mom got it into her head that Dad and Mary Lou could not have a good relationship because he was gone during her infancy. This is something I heard from Mom for as long as I can remember. She said it to Mary Lou and Dad as well. In truth, it was the relationship between *Mom* and Mary Lou that was abysmal. By the time Mary Lou was a teenager, she was both beautiful and stormy. She left home at sixteen to be with her boyfriend, who had joined the Marines. When they returned, they married. It was within weeks of her seventeenth birthday. She and Arne—still married—raised two sons, living most of their married life in the suburbs south of Seattle. While they were geographically close to Mom and Dad, the relationship was distant.

As I sat sheltered in the somewhat overheated living room of my elderly Aunt Dagny, I reflected on my own painful relationship with Mary Lou in the past year. We had been close after we became adults. But the recent strain in her relationship with Mother was putting a strain on our relationship as well. Mary Lou would call me up and swear that Mother was stark raving mad. I lived 300 miles away. I couldn't tell. Mary Lou and Mother had never gotten along. Mary Lou told me, for example, that Mom kept calling her up and asking her to go to an aerobics class with her. Mary Lou was—and is—far from the aerobics-class type. She would tell Mother that she wasn't interested and why. Then Mother, paying no attention to Mary Lou's wants and needs, would ask again. To Mary Lou, it felt as if she were being pressured. Looking back, I can see that these episodes may have been early memory lapses. By the end of 1985, Mary Lou's relationship with her parents was irreparably strained. It had always been fragile, and during this time, it simply was breaking into pieces. As a defense, Mom and Dad decided that *Mary Lou* was the one who was crazy. Upset and depressed about this, Mother couldn't unravel it, couldn't straighten it out. She grieved over it.

Dad would have said that Mary Lou was the source of any unhappiness Mother felt. But Mary Lou, once again, was only a symptom of a much larger underlying problem. And by this time, she was so hurt and angry that if anyone had dared ask her if her mother was happy, she would have responded that she couldn't have cared less.

In a mirror opposite of Mary Lou's relationship with our parents, our brothers, Tom and John, lived farthest from Mom and Dad and enjoyed the closest relationships with them. John, although born third in the family, was the first-born son. John was just two years younger than I. As a young boy, John was fascinated by Native Americans and their cultures. He loved to hunt and fish, loved the out-of-doors. He often said that someday he'd live with the Indians and live off the land. John came of age in the heart of the Viet Nam War. Dad had some connections that got John into the Coast Guard after high school, whereupon he was sent to the North Pole on an ice cutter. This experience made a reader of John. I think it may have turned him into a writer as well, if he had made one more trip up there. His letters to me while I was in college were deep and philosophical—and full of his hatred of the Coast Guard and ice! When John finished his tour of duty, he went on to school, graduating with a degree in finance.

John married Denise while he was still in college. After graduation they lived in Seattle and then moved to Northern Idaho, just across the Washington border. Denise was part Cherokee. She and John settled into a cabin on Hayden Lake and John got involved in real estate and timber lands. It made me laugh to see the way that he was realizing his childhood dream.

John and Denise were close to Mom and Dad. John is like Mother's side of the family in disposition. I think he reminded her of her father and oldest brother. All had a sensitive, serious side and their humor was dry—not goofy like the man she had married. John and Dad often hunted and fished together. Mother and Denise would go out and pick fruit or shop on these trips. Though John and Denise did not have children until they had been married about ten years, their children were closest, also, to our parents. They visited Seattle often, staying with Mom and Dad.

While not a man of many words, John's words are always well-chosen. Like Dad, he has never been one to delve into the psychology of things. Had Aunt Dagny asked John if his mother was happy, he would have said, "Yes." He brought out the best in her, and that is the face of her that he saw.

My youngest brother, Tom, lived with Mom and Dad until he was nearly thirty. He was addicted to cocaine and alcohol, something Mary Lou, John, and I all individually spoke to our parents about. We all gave the same message. Allowing Tom to live at home well into his twenties was enabling his addictions. The message fell on deaf ears. Tom sank ever deeper into the abyss. I was closest to Tom when we were very young. He had asthma from the time he was born and later a bone disease that kept him bedridden for a year. Still, he had the sweetest disposition and a kind humor. Like Dad, he could use humor to brighten any day. He could manipulate a smile from a frown with a single word. During all the drinking years, it was Tom who could coax Mom into laughter. She was very close to him and not able to let go. It broke my heart to see him forever at home, losing ground at a time when he needed to be growing into manhood.

When Tom was around thirty, he moved to Alaska. He'd been up there a time or two before, always returning to Seattle. This time he stayed long enough to run into the kind of trouble that put him before a judge who offered two options. He could get sober and get help, or he could go to jail. Somehow he had just enough gray matter left in his fried brain to choose the first.

As I sat with Aunt Dagny facing her question, I knew that Tom's answer, even after months of work in recovery, would have been, "Happiness? What's that?"

When I heard about Tom getting help from my comfortable home in suburban Spokane, where my two little girls attended a private school and took piano lessons, I sat down and wept for joy. The Good Lord had reached down into the abyss and rescued my little brother.

Speaking of God's hand from Heaven, I'd had a special friend in an older woman named Ruthie who lived across the street from us on Beacon Hill. Ruthie had heart disease, and I actually lived with her half the time for over two years when her husband, a railroad engineer, traveled. I tended Ruthie, as she tended me. I cooked and cleaned for her. I even had my own bedroom at her house. She called me "Hollywood" and thought I was hot stuff. Ruthie remained my closest confidante until she died a few years after our move to the suburbs. She had only met my new boyfriend, Ralph, once—and she told me to hang on to him.

This was during the time when everything was falling apart at home. I remember many dates with Ralph where I would just sit and cry because my home life was such a mess. He had no way of understanding. He was just a good listener. I must have been a barrel of fun as a date.

After high school I moved across town to the University of Washington, where I lived on campus. In contrast to high school when my family had been a huge and unhappy part of my life, at college it hardly existed. Dad drove me to the dorm where he dropped me off at the curb with my belongings. That was the closest anyone in my family ever came to visiting me in three years. I went home for holidays, and there were occasional phone calls to Mom. I talked often with Mary Lou and went out to visit her and her family whenever I could get a ride there. I got a few letters from John when he was in the Coast Guard.

After Ralph and I married, we lived three miles from my parents in the home Ralph was raised in. They never saw the inside of this home either, though I did invite them. A year later, Ralph and I moved across the state to Spokane.

Mother always felt I was too sensitive, too caring. Until I was a teacher, I believed her. Then I realized that being sensitive was an asset. I came to believe that it wasn't possible to be "too sensitive" or to care too deeply, any more that it was possible to be too pretty or too capable.

After teaching a few years, I "retired" to start a family. One wintry day, after driving six hours, we arrived at Mom and Dad's with a cranky baby, which made me anxious with worry for my little Heather. Then Mother started in with the over-sensitivity speech. But she did not get far this time. I stopped her cold by saying, "And if you can't be sensitive and care for your own child, Mother, who in this world do you care for?" It was a double-edged question; *I* felt uncared for by *her*. She never bothered me about my "over-sensitivity" again. It was ironic that her life would depend one day upon my capacity to sense her needs and to care for her.

Our Janelle was born shortly after a transfer back to the Seattle area. I was ill after Janelle was born, suffering from fifteen different infections in six months. From Dad, there was nothing, no real communication of any kind. He distanced himself, I guess. From The Doctor Agnes, K.E., there were occasional questions wondering if I needed help. When I said I did, she let me know how she hated to drive on the freeway. Or in the rain. This was hard to take from a woman who had gone to South Dakota two days after Janelle was born and had gotten herself to Norway a couple of years earlier. It fit into a larger, long-term pattern. When I got well, it was a time of deep disillusionment and grief for me. I nearly left my young family, wondering if families weren't an exercise in futility.

It was time to squarely face this problem. I bitterly confronted Mom and Dad with the fact that I understood now that I could fall off the face of the earth, and they wouldn't much care, certainly not enough to drive across town. If they really wanted any kind of a relationship with me, however, they would at least have to pretend occasionally to care, because I also now knew that I had absolutely nothing to lose. Mother cried in response to this and was genuinely sorry. Dad said he was too old to change; the relationship was over. I'm sure he expected me to "come around" but I honestly and deeply meant what I had said. It took him some time, but eventually it was he who "came around."

That time was my Valley of the Shadow of Death. It is only the hand of God that can bring one through the Valley, and that was my experience. When it was over, I knew three things. I knew I loved and wanted my family of Ralph, Heather, and Janelle more than life itself. No one could love them more than I could love them. Second, I knew that to be whole, I had to love and forgive my parents. No matter how I was treated, to stop loving them would be giving in to something very wrong. This conscious decision came at a greater cost than I ever imagined at the time. Finally, I had to leave my past in the past and not allow it to poison my future; I had to go forward and leave the rubble and the Valley behind me.

This was a pivotal time in my life. There were things I didn't know, didn't understand about it until later. I have come to understand that it is harder to lose people in life than it is in death. For example, to have a husband walk out after twenty years of marriage would be harder to bear than his death after the same period of time. There is not only the loss of him to bear, but also the rejection. Similarly, I grieved the loss of my parents at a time when they were still living. It was a thorough grieving. When I was done, it was over, and never would I grieve the loss of them like that again.

But I have also come to believe that I would never have been emotion-ally healthy without going through the Valley and coming—by conscious choice—out of it. My whole concept and definition of love was revolution-ized in this process. We often think of love as an emotion. The love I committed to was active, not emotional. Having been on the receiving end of inactive "love," I had decided that love without action did not exist. It was empty love—a contradiction in terms. So when I committed to loving, it was a commitment to action, not to a warm, fuzzy feeling. I committed to staying in relationship, to civility, to helping when needed, to being included in family events.

Another thing I did not understand was that in finishing the grieving process, it left a part of me emotionally detached. This odd combination of committing to love and being emotionally detached (at least temporarily) actually turned out to be an asset when in later years my parents needed help.

Certainly I did not know that I'd spend years on a road called Alzheimer's Disease, and that it would change me even more.

By the time Janelle was a year and a half old, Ralph was facing some disillusionment of his own. He quit his job, sold our home, and moved the four of us back to Spokane. We settled back into the familiar suburbs we'd lived in before.

Now our girls were in elementary school and were having a high old time with their father as I was on this short trip to visit my Aunt Dagny.

In that close living room she leaned forward a little to study my response. "Do you think your mother is happy?" she asked me.

Without a moment's hesitation, I said, "No."

Chapter 2

Catching a Cloud
1982-85

The Doctor, as we often called Mother for short, was born in 1916, so in the early 1980s she was in her late sixties; Dad was a few years younger. They were mostly retired. Dad still dabbled in real estate; The Doctor continued to do some bookkeeping for a friend.

Their brick home in Shorewood on the south rim of Seattle overlooking Puget Sound had an airy quality to it. Large picture windows graced the whole front of the house for a panoramic view. From here they could watch ships pass, follow ferries on their routine voyages, and see the fog lift in the morning. Vashon Island was in the distance. The patio in the back of the house was bordered by a little wood and enjoyed cool breezes of the salty air that flowed off the water. Inside the house the walls were the warmth of wood or an off-white that just hinted at the pastels The Doctor loved. This was the home they had moved into with their four children after leaving Beacon Hill.

In contrast to their home and its peaceful qualities, their lives were in constant motion. They always enjoyed a busy social life, and this intensified now that they were no longer burdened with child-rearing and work. Hard times were behind them. This was a time to enjoy.

Even though Mom and Dad had strained relationships with both daughters, this has to be viewed as a flaw, not as a characteristic. Mother was characteristically warm, loving, and helpful to people. Before the age of therapists, she was often sought out by her friends and neighbors for her wise counsel. Dad never knew a stranger.

Good to a fault with their friends, their door was always open. Friends and relatives from far and wide were constantly dropping in for a day or two or a week. Mom and Dad never locked the house unless they were leaving for a week or more. Everyone knew that the key was in an old "snoose" can in the brick planter by the front steps if they happened by and the door *was* locked.

My folks were always on good terms with neighbors who also frequented their home. It was an unusual day when at least three neighbors didn't drop by for a cup of coffee and some chit-chat. One neighbor usually visited in the mornings. Early evenings another neighbor came down the hill, or one of his kids, or one of his kids' kids. The next-door neighbors were in and out all day long. Frequently, Dad would be "allowing" someone to fix his plumbing or re-wire something for him. Perhaps he needed help in the yard or with patching the roof? The motor home might need some adjustment. People loved to help Dad, never noticing that he mostly provided the conversation.

Then there were the bridge clubs. They belonged to a couples' group that got together on Saturday nights. The Doctor also belonged to a women's bridge club. Both of these went back nearly thirty years. Mother belonged to the Lutheran church and sang in the choir from time to time. Dad played poker with buddies in White Center.

And there was the telephone. Dad talked to Homer daily. He also kept in close touch with many other friends and relatives, near and far. People called him about real estate. Should they buy this? Would he sell that? Dad loaned money to just about everyone he knew, so there were calls about one financial transaction after another. The phone was going constantly.

Had this been their only social life, however, I'm sure they would have fainted dead away from the boredom. There was, after all, a whole world *out there* with things to see and do. So they saw and did. They went fishing and dug clams. They camped. They went to Vegas and stayed in hotels. They took the ferry to the San Juan Islands and played bridge; they harvested oysters which The Doctor would crack and eat raw on the beach. They went boating and set out crab pots. They had a place at the ocean, another in the mountains—pieces of land where they could park a trailer or motor home or pitch a tent. They went to reunions in Kansas, checked out Mexico, Hawaii, Canada, and looked up relatives on the East Coast when they were in the neighborhood. Mother said that it didn't matter where they were, there was always someone who knew Dad. They could be in a little drugstore in some far-flung place half way across the country and someone would call out, "Well, Chuck! How the hell *are* you?!" When Dad had a second back surgery, it was sandwiched between a fishing trip with Homer and Betty and the clam season. Saying that my mother and father were enjoying an active retirement would have been understating it. It's no wonder that the first glimmer of Alzheimer's was lost in the commotion.

The Doctor was a product of her Scandinavian, South Dakota upbringing. She was a good housekeeper from the "cleanliness is next to Godliness" school of thought. Denial was her chief coping mechanism. Complaining was a taboo. And she was seldom depressed, believing that one should just get up and get going when feeling blue. Apart from that, however, The Doctor was cheerful and enthusiastic on her own, choosing to be happy amid nearly anything. For example, Mom had hammer toes, perhaps the result of poverty and poor-fitting shoes as a child. As a result, on at least eight toes she had *multiple* corns. She treated these regularly, but they always came back. Having never heard a complaint, I didn't know they hurt until I was an adult, and a podiatrist told me they were painful. What I did know was that good fitting shoes were extremely important, right up there with cleanliness. While she could have been quietly sedentary with this problem, she was not. The Doctor's idea of a treat was a brisk *walk* outdoors.

Finding the beginning of Alzheimer's is like trying to catch a cloud. One is never sure when it is found. While hindsight may be 20/20, it doesn't help much when trying to discern something barely there. Who can find the true beginning of Alzheimer's? We all have moments of forgetfulness, for example. So which ones signify the onset of disease? We all have times of malaise, small depressions, and times of upset. When are these symptoms of something larger? From 1982 to 1985 there were traces of Alzheimer's, I believe, in Mother. Any one thing by itself was inconsequential. Taken together as a whole, they began to form just an impression that something was not quite right.

There was the family reunion in Spokane in 1982 when The Doctor didn't recognize Pee Wee. The loss of tact with her sisters. The sense that some in the family had that Mom was unhappy. The problems Mary Lou reported.

All her life The Doctor was very determined to make the best of things, to put on a happy face. The years of alcoholism had been glued together with her determination. In the early- to mid-1980s, she even told one of her dearest friends, Joan Reiter, that she literally got up each day and consciously put on a smile. She told Joan what a horrible thing it would be to lose one's mind, that she would hate to be in an accident or have a stroke and end up helpless with no control. She feared becoming a burden. Joan remembers the conversation because Mom got lost driving back from Joan's home that same day.

Once when my Aunt Babe and Uncle Larry visited Mom and Dad, driving all the way from El Paso, there was no coffee in the house. In a Scandinavian home this would be like not having your head attached to your neck—inconceivable. Hours later, the coffee turned up in some remote spot. Everyone thought The Doctor had played a joke. In hindsight, it might have been that Mother put the coffee away in an unlikely spot and then couldn't find it. It is not uncommon for people with early Alzheimer's to seem to be hiding things, when in reality, they are just forgetting where they put them—and they have put them in the wrong place!

Other characteristics began to change. I visited Mom a few times a year. I was noticing that the house was often messy. Over time it seemed to get messier. I asked Mary Lou about it, and she assured me that it was because she and I weren't around to clean for Mom anymore. Having a more distant perspective, I wasn't so sure.

In 1984 Dad had seven by-passes done on his heart. I left Ralph and my girls at home and spent several days with my parents. I stayed with Mom while Dad was in the hospital and then stayed a couple of days after Dad got home. I noticed nothing in particular about Mother. I was more focused on Dad, of course, but generally Mom seemed to be functioning normally.

But by the end of 1985, Dad was noticing that something was wrong with Mother because he was frequently asking me if I thought she looked thin. When I said I thought she looked about the same he would drop it. But every time I saw my parents for at least a full year after the heart surgery,

Dad would ask again, "How do you think your mother looks?"

By the end of 1985, my parents' relationship with Mary Lou was broken. And The Doctor had sent out Christmas cards *twice.* Some friends still didn't get a card.

Chapter 3

1986

No one remembers the exact day Mother fell on her way out of the suburban library she frequented. It was in the spring. She hit her head and banged up her face pretty badly. Dad would probably mark that event as the beginning of Mother's Alzheimer's. He sent her to the doctor's office more than once about it and complained to me that he was not sure she remembered why she was at the doctor's office in the first place. I thought this was just Mother's way—a bit of denial and a lifelong habit of putting a happy face on things. The physician would ask her how she was, and she'd say, "I'm great!" Babe later told me that around the time of the fall Mom told her she'd had periods of blackouts—times when she remembered nothing. She *knew* something was wrong, even if the rest of us were just wondering about it. It was early in the summer of 1986 that I had visited my Aunt Dagny and she had asked me, "Do you think your mother is happy?" Neither of us could pinpoint a cause for unhappiness.

August of 1986 brought Mom's 70th birthday. A party for her was given at Homer and Betty Schmitt's. They lived in a brick house at the *north* end of Seattle. Their home also had a beautiful view of Puget Sound with a patio in back of the house. The party was on the patio, but there was a little dancing in the kitchen. Dad and Homer were constantly joking back and forth, never failing to give someone a fit of giggles. All the Doctor's longtime friends were there. Pee Wee and Fatty came from Denver and Boise respectively. Aunt Dagny wasn't well enough to make the trip, but Aunt Babe and Uncle Larry came from Texas. It was a great surprise to Mom, and she was thrilled.

In September when my parents came to Spokane for a visit, Mother and

I took a walk together through a nearby pine wood, just the two of us. The Doctor repeated the same conversations over and over during a short half-hour walk. She asked the same questions time and again. When I got back to Dad, I cornered him and told him to get Mom to a doctor and to go in with her, so she couldn't forget anything.

Looking back, it is hard for me to believe how blind I was. But the incidents I've pieced together now were just widely separated events, only traces of a serious problem. To the reader, they seem unnaturally close together. These few incidents happened over a span of four years, and I did not have all the pieces at this early stage. For example, the incident with Mom not recognizing Pee Wee wasn't told to me for years. Babe didn't tell me until years later that Mom had said she was having memory lapses—what she called "blackouts." Mom's friend, Joan, related the incident of getting lost and worrying about losing her mind to me many years later when I told her I was writing about The Doctor. I must admit, I was never able to pin down a problem until the walk and repetitious conversation in Spokane.

Dad did go in with Mother to the doctor. Some tests were done to rule out a stroke. We did not get a definite diagnosis that year, but the physician told Dad that he suspected Alzheimer's. He told Dad if there were any trips he had been putting off, now was the time to go.

Tom's life had turned around quickly after he sought help for his addictions. He married Teri, and by the fall of 1986, they were expecting their first child. Dad and I struggled over what to do about the upcoming birth of Tom and Teri's child. Mom had her heart set on going to Anchorage to be with them when the baby came at the end of November. Since Mom was having times of total clarity and only very occasional periods of forgetfulness, Dad decided to say nothing to Tom and see if Tom even noticed. Tom had been told nothing about Mother except that she had been involved in a fall months earlier and had gone to the doctor to rule out a little stroke.

It was a mistake for Mom to go. Being away from home brought out the worst of symptoms. Mother called Teri "Denise" (her other daughter-in-law) the whole time she was there and drove Tom wild with repeated conversations. Tom called to ask, "What the hell is wrong with Mother?!"

Around this time there had been news reports of a man who shot his wife who had Alzheimer's. Tom let me know his sympathies were with the man.

One of the things that began to develop at this early stage was a symbiotic relationship with Dad. As Dad's physical health declined, Mom's mind declined. Dad could tell Mom what to do. He could go through the steps of getting something done with her. Mom could do it. As the disease progressed, Mom could not think or choose a course of action. Dad became less and less able to do physical things. But as a team, they operated pretty well for several years. Dad was the brain and The Doctor, wonderfully fit and exercising daily, was the brawn. If the bridge club was being hosted, for example, Dad might say, "Let's go downstairs and get the card table." Together they would go to the basement, and when they got there it was Dad who knew why they were there! He'd give The Doctor the card table and perhaps he'd take a chair. Together they would walk back up and put these in the living room. Then down they'd go again, with The Doctor returning with two chairs, while Dad carried one. This symbiosis continued and deepened as time went on. It was fascinating to watch the natural development of it between the two of them.

By the end of 1986 the immediate family knew there was a definite problem. Homer and Betty had been told that there was a problem. My parents' closest and lifelong friends, they also were noticing some different behaviors. No one else really knew. Dad was afraid that, if he told people, they would be uncomfortable, and he would lose his friends. When Mother was in groups of three or more people, she could easily hide it. In situations where conversation flowed along, her symptoms did not appear at all. She still played cards fairly well, and she still paid the bills. She still functioned in her home with meals and upkeep, except it kept getting messier. Of course if anyone wanted to know how she was, she would tell them she was wonderful. *Couldn't* be better!

None of us, friends or family, had any idea of the magnitude of the problems we were facing. Little did we know that the kernel of a solution was buried in a family story I'd entertained Aunt Dagny with on my visit that summer.

After we left Beacon Hill, Mother had worked for years for a man named Richard Yarrington. He owned a funeral home on the outskirts of the south end of Seattle. Of course, Mom had prior experience in the funeral business. She had a childhood laced with acting as mourner among her pioneer siblings on the plains of South Dakota. For Mr. Yarrington she was bookkeeper and office manager. She also got to know many a bereaved widow and widower, undoubtedly because she was such a sympathetic listener. She would naturally cry. She came home regularly with a high-pitched lecture to us about how to behave when she died. It went something like this: "You do not honor a person when they die by fighting over his *things*. I am going to leave *every*thing I have to charity just so you won't have *any*thing to fight over when I am gone! Why, I see these people who have lost their dear mother and all that they *think* about is whether Susie gets the hutch or whether Steven should have it. I won't have my family *fight*ing over my *things*! Steven won't speak to Susie any more and WHY?! Well it's all about MONEY!" She could go on like this for quite some time, talking about people we didn't know and driving home her point. My aunt, facing her own mortality, chuckled and agreed heartily.

Unfortunately, Mom was partly "gone" years before she actually died. Scattered over three states, her family had suffered through alcoholism, bankruptcy, divorce proceedings, drug addiction, serious illnesses, and rifts. There was a husband who had "beaten" alcoholism in a John Wayne sort of way, that is, without help or much analysis. There was a daughter, Mary Lou, who lived near her with whom she had a broken relationship. Another daughter stayed in touch from the other side of the state, somewhat as detached emotionally as she was physically. She had two sons who had established themselves in two other states. John was in Idaho. Tom—who was crawling out of addiction—was in Alaska. And she had a disease hiding in her future that would force her dependency upon this unlikely group as it threatened to tear all memory from her ever curious mind and to rip all dignity from her.

But we had been well-coached. When Mother "left" us, we had to figure out how to pull together, and we knew it had better be without fighting. We had to take good care of The Doctor. This is *her* story.

Chapter 4

Alzheimer's Disease

Alzheimer's Disease takes some time to accurately diagnose. From the beginning, Mother's physician told Dad that this was what he was suspecting.

Dad couldn't bear to think of Mother having Alzheimer's. He'd heard a few horror stories, read a little, been told a little, seen a little on TV. That was enough. He could bear to know no more. He told me to read up on it. Then I could tell him what he needed to know as we went along. Since denial is a coping mechanism commonly used not only by victims of Alzheimer's, but also by their caregivers, Dad didn't even want to believe at first that The Doctor really had this disease. He himself went in and out of being able to believe it.

I spent the better part of one summer reading books and articles on Alzheimer's. I went through a few medical books and some periodicals written on the subject. I also read *The Loss of Self* by Donna Cohen and Carl Eisdorfer, "Alzheimer's Disease: Report of the Secretary of Health and Human Services Task Force on Alzheimer's Disease," and *Alzheimer's: A Caregiver's Guide and Sourcebook* by Howard Gruetzner.

I went so far as to copy pages from two of these regarding the course of the disease. Then, when I saw the symptoms appear in Mom, I wrote the dates in the margin to the side. I continued this practice for the rest of Mom's life. Naturally, as time went along, articles appeared in newspapers and magazines. The subject became much more popular. I tried to keep current as the disease progressed in Mom.

I learned that Alzheimer's Disease (A.D.) was first described by a German physician, Alois Alzheimer, in 1906. It is not a "new" disease. It is a disease in which the brain cells are destroyed. As it moves through the brain, memory, the ability to talk meaningfully, emotion, behavior, and motor control are all affected. A.D. may begin with recent memory loss and end with virtually all memory lost. At some stages of the disease, the patient suffers mental illness, generally called dementia, which literally means "out of one's mind." It manifests itself in the form of depression, paranoia (unreasonable fears), and delusions or hallucinations. The person loses control over emotion and may fly into rages, becoming violent or hysterical. In the early stages, this may manifest itself simply as the loss of tact and/or depression. In the middle stages, emotions are more violently expressed as rages, paranoia, and/or hysteria. Near the end of the disease, delusions and a break with reality altogether may occur.

Motor control is also affected. Alzheimer's victims will fall, have difficulty with buttons and zippers, eventually lose control of bodily functions, lose the ability to swallow, and even "forget" how to walk.

Alzheimer's disease comes in two forms. The less common form has an age of onset as early as 45-55 years old. In this form, the disease may progress more rapidly, and the patient has a life expectancy of three to five years. This form is called "early-onset Alzheimer's." It is sometimes called "familial Alzheimer's" because it is genetically linked. Early onset Alzheimer's makes up about 10% of all Alzheimer's cases.

The more common form of the disease is age-related and occurs after age 65. Life expectancy for this form typically is seven to ten years or more, and it may also have genetic links. I have read varying statistics, but generally it is uncommon in people under 55 years old. By age 70, one in twelve people has Alzheimer's. By age 80, the chance of having Alzheimer's is as high as one in three. "Forty-seven percent of those over 85 have the disease" (Marmor, 1995).

Alzheimer's is a *degenerative* disease. That means that one who has it will get measurably worse over time. If Aunt Sue is forgetful and a bit off balance mentally and a doctor once said, "Oh, it's probably Alzheimer's," chances are good that it is NOT Alzheimer's unless over the course of six months or a year Aunt Sue worsens steadily. If Aunt Sue "has been like this for years" then there is something else wrong with Aunt Sue because Alzheimer's is degenerative. A victim of Alzheimer's does not stay the same over time.

Alzheimer's is also a *terminal* disease. People do die of its effects. It is considered the fourth leading cause of death for adults, after heart disease, cancer, and stroke (Nadler-Moodie and Wilson, 1998). However, since it most often strikes older people and progresses slowly, many victims frequently die of something else first. They die of the same things that other older people die of—heart disease, stroke, pneumonia, and so forth.

Much of the research done with Alzheimer's focuses on the medical side of things—causes, ways to diagnose, and medications for example.

The cause of the vast majority of Alzheimer's disease is unknown, except for the genetic mutation found with early onset Alzheimer's and a genetic predisposition for some of the rest. It is known that the brain of any Alzheimer's victim is riddled with tangles and plaques. Tangles are protein inside the damaged brain cells. Plaques are debris found outside of dead nerve cells in the brain. It is not known whether the tangles and plaques are the cause of Alzheimer's or the result of it.

There are many theories about causes of Alzheimer's. Some research is focusing on environmental factors. Aluminum appears to play a role in the disease because high aluminum content is found in the brain of Alzheimer's victims. Here again, it is not known whether this is a cause or an effect. Zinc is another mineral under investigation. A link between electromagnetic fields and Alzheimer's is under study.

There have been theories that the disease is caused by a bacteria or virus, as yet undiscovered. Recently there have been headlines about the relationship between estrogen and Alzheimer's. Another study looked at the risk of developing Alzheimer's and the use of nonsteroidal anti-inflammatory drugs, such as ibuprofen. Some of the latest research is considering multiple factors that may trigger the disease. Medical investigations regarding Alzheimer's have been around for a number of years.

Alzheimer's is an incurable disease—so far. There is no known cure; however, there are drugs to help alleviate Alzheimer's symptoms, slow its progress, and improve memory for some patients in the earlier stages of the disease. There are medicines that help Alzheimer's patients with the mental illness that comes with the disease. There are medications for depression, paranoia, and agitation. Some say herbal remedies such as ginkgo biloba help with the early memory losses. So far, all the available drugs treat the *symptoms* of Alzheimer's. They neither cure nor prevent the disease.

Research on functioning focuses on the behavioral and care side of the disease. Finding ways to help Alzheimer's victims use their remaining abilities in order to make themselves as independent as possible for as long as possible is a more recent area of research. The University of Washington, for example, is trying to find ways to extend the functioning of Alzheimer's victims.

The Alzheimer's Association lists these ten warning signs of a dementing illness:

> memory loss that affects job skills
> difficulty performing familiar tasks
> problems with language
> disorientation of time and place
> poor or decreased judgment
> problems with abstract thinking
> misplacing things
> changes in mood behavior
> changes in personality
> loss of initiative

Other information is available from The Alzheimer's Association, including the location of hundreds of support groups around the country. Their toll free phone number is 1-800-272-3900. They can be reached by mail at 919 North Michigan Avenue, Suite 1000, Chicago, IL 60611-1676. The Alzheimer's home page address is http://www.alz.org/.

For The Doctor Agnes, K.E., our first step was to get a diagnosis. Diagnosis of Alzheimer's is a complex process. In the United States, because of ethical reasons, brain biopsy is done only for suspected cancer. In parts of Europe, physicians actually biopsy the brain to diagnose Alzheimer's. Finding ways to better diagnose the disease is an area of intense, on-going research.

To diagnose Alzheimer's in the U.S., other possible causes for symptoms *must* be ruled out first. There are many things that cause Alzheimer's-like symptoms. A variety of causes exist for mental illness, for example. Diabetes, hypothyroidism, strokes, and even some medications all can produce symptoms similar to Alzheimer's.

Once all other possibilities have been ruled out, then there is over a 90% likelihood that the patient with the symptoms has Alzheimer's, though other, more rare diseases are still a possibility.

Next the patient undergoes mental testing over a period of six months to a year. Because Alzheimer's is degenerative, it changes over time. By undergoing mental tests periodically, and comparing them, an almost certain diagnosis can be made.

The diagnosis for Mom took a year. She went through a number of tests including a CAT scan, blood work, and so forth. She was given a mental abilities test that was repeated in six months and again in a year. Her diagnosis was confirmed at that time.

Mother was a member of Group Health Cooperative. They were doing a study with the University of Washington's Medical School and asked The Doctor if she wanted to be part of it. She was still able to reason while she was undergoing diagnosis. Her main problems were with short term memory, not logic. The idea of being part of research, of contributing to health and medicine, was right up her alley. Never mind the fact that she was still denying there was anything wrong with her!

Once I'd done the reading, friends and family began to ask me about Alzheimer's. What did we called Alzheimer's before it was widely known? Part of the answer is that people didn't live as long, and the vast majority of Alzheimer's cases are of the age-related type. I can't tell the number of times people have said to me, "Isn't Alzheimer's just what we used to call senility?" The answer is "No." Alzheimer's is an illness. Senility is the dulling of the senses that occurs as we age. It is part of the normal aging process. We all become a little more forgetful as we get older. John's wife, Denise, had a grandmother who lived to be in her nineties. Denise said toward the end that her grandmother was somewhat senile. She moved slowly, and her reactions, even in thought, had slowed. Her hearing and eyesight were dulled. How different that was from what Mom was experiencing!

One evening my husband, Ralph, and I went out for dinner with a group from our church. On the way in a bus we got to talking with a couple, and I mentioned Mom and her Alzheimer's.

The woman said, "Isn't Alzheimer's just what we used to call . . . "

I was thinking, "Oh, here we go again."

Then she said, ". . . madness?"

I nearly jumped out of my seat. "Yes!" I said. "We used to refer to that crazy old lady down the street! We used to talk of an older person as being 'off his rocker!'"

Alzheimer's isn't just part of the aging process. It is a disease. We don't know the cause, and we don't have a cure. We do know that it kills brain cells and that it moves from one part of the brain to another, leaving destruction in its wake. People used to be ashamed of mental illness, dementia, what we now know are diseases of the brain. If a family member was afflicted, one never spoke of it. The family member might be put in an insane asylum. It wasn't discussed publicly. This is another reason why people never heard of A.D., or thought it to be uncommon.

After much research and caring for The Doctor both directly and indirectly for a number of years, I came to disagree with the experts on two points. First, many experts say that victims of Alzheimer's don't know that they have it. This is inconsistent with the idea that the dominant way of dealing with Alzheimer's is denial. Denial of what? If there weren't awareness on some level, there could be no denial. Yet denial is mentioned frequently in the literature as a dominant coping mechanism. Gruetzner noted that of all the different kinds of senile dementia, Alzheimer's is the only one where the victims *try to hide* the symptoms of illness. A person does not try to hide something if he is unaware that it is there! It amazed everyone who knew her how well The Doctor could hide her illness. I'm sure that she worked at it. In addition to the incident where Mom spoke to her friend, Joan, about the fear of losing her mind, I will relate a number of events about The Doctor that further strengthen the observation that she *knew* there was something wrong with her mind.

Second, it is widely advised by the experts that, particularly in the later stages of this disease, the patient should be institutionalized. Nursing homes have a financial interest in keeping control of Alzheimer's patients because ". . . 80% of elderly nursing home residents have a psychiatric disorder; most of those have Alzheimer's" (Brownlee, 1991). There's big money in taking care of an aging population. But many Alzheimer's patients do not even need the expensive skilled nursing care that nursing homes provide. Many need only custodial care. They need someone to bathe, feed, dress, walk, and watch them. Because they lack the ability to communicate their needs, they are like infants. I found that one-on-one care is best. The nature of an institution, like a nursing home or Alzheimer's care center, is shifts of people, three shifts a day, and different shifts on weekends. This is confusing for an Alzheimer's patient. There can be no ownership of an individual's care. There can be no continuity of care, no comforting familiarity of care. Like the confusion of taking a trip and being away from home, institutional care can actually be detrimental.

Foster care, on the other hand, provides a solution for all of these needs. Foster care, known also as "adult family care," takes place in a regular home, in a regular neighborhood. The patient lives with only a few other people and has only one or two caregivers. Of course the home is modified in some ways. There may be ramps instead of steps, fenced and locked back yards and decks, special intercom systems, and so on. In my state, Washington, foster care is licensed to assure certain standards of safety and care. Some foster homes do provide skilled nursing care; others can have visiting nurses come in a few times a week. Some also provide day care. Furthermore, foster care is often less expensive. In my area it costs *half* of what Alzheimer's care in a nursing home or Alzheimer's care facility costs. In addition, it is so much more pleasant for the patient and for the visiting friends and family.

Unfortunately, few physicians are familiar with foster care as an option. Very few have been to a foster care facility. Public health nurses, social service agencies, and Alzheimer's support groups can be good local sources of information on foster care. Some foster care homes will also let the Alzheimer's victim and his or her spouse move in together. Foster care is a wonderful alternative for Alzheimer's patients, and I found scant mention of it in the literature.

Information on A.D. is now much more widely available than it was when I first began to learn of it. There are also many more chapters of The Alzheimer's Association, which can provide wonderful support for caregivers and victims alike.

Alzheimer's disease follows a pattern. Stages of the disease have been identified. The Doctor Agnes, K.E., was only beginning her walk down this long road as I spent the summer reading to help my dad. Meanwhile, Mom was still traveling, playing bridge, enjoying her home and friends. But inwardly she was fighting depression and a growing anxiety.

The Late Confusional Stage

This stage manifests a general worsening of symptoms begun in the first stage. As memory worsens, the person has difficulty following a conversation, retaining the thread of a story whether read or watched on television. He or she is not able to keep up with current events in the news. Making plans and decisions becomes difficult. The person becomes more anxious, more confused, and sometimes more angry or depressed. Denying there is a problem, he or she does not welcome help. The ability to drive worsens, although short, familiar trips to the store, to church, and so on are still possible. Because recent memory is more impaired, the person may speak more of events in the distant past that are still quite clear. Simple, routine tasks are still easily accomplished, but the ability to pay bills and keep track of finances, play cards, and similar, more complicated tasks is diminished. Because the victim's abilities are diminishing, he or she may become more self-absorbed and less able to see or meet needs of others. At this point there is usually the development of a caregiver, someone who tries to help the person who denies the need. The caregiver at this stage is both unwanted and unappreciated. It's a tough role and it gets no easier.

Repetitive behaviors (perseverations) are common throughout Alzheimer's. In the earlier stages, this is most noticeable in speech. The person repeats the same phrases, thoughts, or questions. Later perseverations include behaviors.

There is overlap between the stages of any disease. One set of symptoms does not abruptly stop and another start. Rather, symptoms intensify. One set gradually gives way to another. The primary difference between the first two stages of Alzheimer's is that in stage one the symptoms are subtle; in stage two they are more obvious to others (Gruetzner, 1988).

Chapter 5

1987

Mother did not enter stage two just because we rang in a new year. Certainly her symptoms were obvious to me by then and to Tom and Teri when The Doctor came to "help" with their new baby at the end of 1986. For the sake of clarity and organization, and to give the reader a sense of the time The Doctor spent in each stage, I'll break them down by year. Of course each person will progress through the stages at an individual rate. Factors like general health come into play, for example.

After Christmas, 1986, Mom and Dad drove to Las Vegas as was their annual habit. Dad liked to gamble, liked the shows, liked the climate, and loved all the people. Mom really didn't like Las Vegas at all, but she always went, spending time with Dad's sister, Ethel. The two of them would go to church together and, as a counterpoint to their husbands, keep regular hours. Auntie Ethel, as sweet and decent a woman as God ever graced upon His earth, loved her "little" brother Bud with her whole heart, in spite of his colorful ways. It was Auntie Ethel who tended to the basic needs of the group as they ventured each year to Las Vegas. For a couple of years, Auntie Ethel had worried about The Doctor. She thought that she might be drinking, because she went off by herself and sat in a corner with the slot machines and a drink and often seemed disoriented. Auntie Ethel was also hurt that Mom wasn't as nice to her as she had once been. Still Auntie Ethel faithfully made the annual trek to Las Vegas this year. Around the first of March, Auntie Ethel and Uncle Harold would go south to their home, while Mom and Dad went north to theirs.

My husband Ralph had been transferred to Portland, Oregon, effective the first of the year. I had to stay in Spokane until our house sold. One

February weekend I drove Heather and Janelle over the wintry mountains to Seattle to stay in Mom and Dad's vacated house. Ralph drove up from Portland to meet us there. We let ourselves in using the key that was hidden in the snuff box in the front planter. When we got in the house I noticed first that the iron was still on. Then I saw that the electric blanket on Mom's side of her bed was still on—*and had been for over a month*. Needless to say, I let Dad know he was lucky the house hadn't burned down.

We moved across the state in March of that year and rented a house in the small town of Battle Ground fifteen miles north of Portland, Oregon, on the Washington side of the Columbia River. Mom and Dad came down to Battle Ground for Easter, and we showed them various properties that we were considering buying. Dad fell in love with a wooded five-acre piece with a creek running through it. The Doctor liked it too. It was the one we eventually bought. We had invited our pastor and his wife to Easter dinner also, and we took turns playing bridge together after dinner. This was something The Doctor Agnes, K.E., retained as an ability long after the books said she would be able.

Taking the advice of Mom's physician, Mom and Dad went on a couple of trips in 1987. They went to Australia with Homer and Betty. It was a trip Dad had long wanted to do. While Homer and Dad had a good time visiting topless beaches and taking plenty of pictures, there were some strains because of Mom's worsening condition. Betty said that Mom took the "insulting" banter between Homer and Dad seriously. For example, if the four of them were walking down the street after a day of sightseeing, looking for a restaurant for dinner, Homer might look over at Dad and say in mock sympathy, "It sure is too bad that you're not wearing a jacket, or we could go in that restaurant across the street. Just look at you—they'll never let you in!" Betty would laugh and point out that Homer was also wearing slacks and a sports shirt. Dad, always serious when it came to dinner, would tell Homer with a pitying expression, "Homer, I could *charm* my way into any establishment on this island. It is *you* who can't go in." Normally Mom would be part of this too, informing the fellas that she and Betty did not need the likes of *them* to have dinner! On this trip, however, The Doctor just stood there looking sad, perhaps even to the point of crying. People were saying unkind things to each other, after all, and to make things worse, they would all go without dinner. Homer, Betty, and Dad would then have to comfort Mom, and tell her it was only a joke. It was a time when they all began to realize that the wonderful foursome they had been for so many years was coming apart.

My Aunt Dagny died that year, and Mom and Dad went to Idaho Falls for her funeral. Mother came home and told me how shocked the whole family was at Pee Wee's new boyfriend, who was black. Pee Wee felt she needed her boyfriend for comfort and support. Mom said it didn't bother *her* that Pee Wee's boyfriend was black, but she thought it was upsetting to Dagny as she was dying to have this going on. Mom was still able to make a judgment about some issues.

The Doctor Agnes, K.E., could still decide things, make judgments, and speak her mind, giving us a window of opportunity for learning what kind of care she wanted in the future. A tentative diagnosis of Alzheimer's had been made, but she was still capable of determining her course. For example, she could have told her children that she didn't want to live with them. She told both Auntie Ethel and Aunt Babe as much. She could have executed a living will with very little help, but we didn't think of it at the time. She did tell Aunt Babe that she never wanted to be in pain, but that she also didn't want to be kept alive as a "vegetable." She also told Babe on an earlier trip to South Dakota that she wouldn't want people to see her if she was "drugged up in a nursing home." We had some ideas about her wishes, but we might have been more direct in our planning. Looking back, I regret that we didn't seize the moment.

Since Mom and Dad were first married, they had always had Thanksgiving dinner with Homer and Betty's family and Betty's sister, Helen, and her family. For over forty years it was the Leonards, the Schmitts, and the Binghams together at Thanksgiving. They took turns hosting it in their homes. Whoever cooked the turkey also did the stuffing, mashed potatoes and gravy. The other two families split the other foods between them to bring to the feast. In 1987, Mother was to bring the pumpkin pies plus some other things to the dinner. First she tried making pumpkin pies as she always did. But they burned or something. Then Dad went out and bought pie shells and a mix for the pies. Another disaster: the pies didn't set. They were too runny after being cooked. So then, Thanksgiving morning, Dad drove all over looking for an open store that still had ready made pumpkin pies. Mom and Dad never hosted Thanksgiving dinner after that. From then on, they were assigned foods like olives, pickles, bread, and beverages to bring.

By the end of 1987, Mom's doctors at Group Health Cooperative had diagnosed her as having Alzheimer's disease. It takes time to pinpoint a diagnosis of Alzheimer's. The patient must be watched and measured for some time after other illnesses have been ruled out. Mother underwent a CAT scan and many other tests when Dad first took her in. Then he was given a tentative diagnosis. Mom's doctor had told him to get his traveling done. Finally—a year later—we had a firm diagnosis. Beyond family and Homer and Betty, most of Mom's friends and neighbors still didn't know.

It still amazes me that Dad never lost his patience with The Doctor—not before her diagnosis or after. She could ask the same question of him a hundred times in the course of an hour or so, and each time he answered her as if it was the first. Once Tom got tired of the same questions over and over again. He continued to answer her in a friendly way; he just made up new and "improved" answers as he went along. Dad chided him for this and told him that Mom was confused enough as it was. Dad would save his short temper for the rest of us. His heart condition was worsening, which didn't help. But he never was anything but gentle and kind to Mom.

Dad had been told that he would be better off not to tell people about Mom's Alzheimer's. I think perhaps Mom's doctor told him this. People might drop away from his social circle when they know about this kind of disease. Dad was such a social creature. He couldn't bear not to have people around him all the time. So he kept his lonely secret, and Mother continued in denial. Her depressions were chalked up to grief over Mary Lou. And so another year passed.

Early Dementia

This stage is marked by increased dependency upon a caregiver. Because the Alzheimer's victim can appear so very normal at times, the caregiver's role is vastly underestimated by neighbors, family, and friends.

Earlier symptoms of the disease intensify still further. Memory gaps are so large that the person may withdraw somewhat socially. He/she may make up things to fill things in. The person's information thus becomes unreliable. It isn't truly lying; the person is not trying to deceive. This is an effort to remain involved in conversation, in life.

The ability to complete a task is diminished. A person may get partially dressed, for example. He or she may begin something and fail to finish it.

Driving in this stage is very dangerous. The person can become lost easily, and reflex ability is slower. Further, the person may over-react in driving situations. This can be a thorny issue for the family. There are tests one can take to demonstrate to the Alzheimer's patient that he or she should not be driving. However, the ability to reason is not terrific at this stage either. Logical, sequential reasoning is becoming impaired.

General orientation of the individual in space and time becomes problematic. The person in this stage of Alzheimer's begins to lose a sense of seasons, time of day, month, direction, place and space. The individual gets lost easily.

Emotional problems develop for a variety of reasons. Alzheimer's itself causes emotional problems as parts of the brain die. A person with Alzheimer's also feels increasingly insecure as memory is affected and confusion about time and space set in. The individual is increasingly suspicious and fearful. Emotionally, he or she is becoming unstable. (Gruetzner, 1988)

Chapter 6

1988-89

Mom and Dad took a side trip down to El Paso from Las Vegas during the winter of 1988. My Aunt Babe had her sister help her fix dinner one night only to find Mom throwing lettuce and other salad fixings out the back door. In The Doctor's back yard in Seattle she had a patio bordered by a little wood. It was her custom to toss things out into the woods to feed the birds and other critters. The Doctor Agnes, K.E., had a whole collection of different birds that came for the various snacks she tossed out. The backyard neighbors looked a little different at my aunt's place in El Paso. Aunt Babe didn't make a fuss over it. She just made another salad. This is a good example, though, of time and place losing meaning for someone with Alzheimer's. Mom functioned better at home, but Dad really needed to travel to keep his sanity.

After they got back to Las Vegas, Dad got pneumonia. Auntie Ethel and Uncle Harold were there to take care of Mom while he was in the hospital. They called my brother John and me to arrange to get Mom and Dad back home. We decided that John and Denise would fly to Las Vegas, play for a day or two, and then drive Mom and Dad home when Dad was up to a trip. I got John and Denise's children, Natalie and Andrew, for the duration. I was taking some graduate level classes at the time and couldn't go to Vegas myself.

In the course of getting this straightened out, Denise called Dad's hospital room in Las Vegas. Mom was with him at the time, as was his physician, so Denise asked to speak to Dad's doctor. She asked about Dad's condition and the doctor was a bit put out or busy or something because he said to Denise, "I have just told all of this to his wife!" To which Denise replied, "But she has Alzheimer's disease and won't remember it to tell me." The doctor, who had probably known Mom for a total of twenty minutes, replied, "She does not!" Still Denise said, "I'd like to hear it from you." He gave Denise the information. All of us felt that it was unethical for that physician to give a diagnosis of a person who was not his own patient. The doctor demonstrated an ignorance of Alzheimer's. We felt he was unethical to contradict a relative who knew Mom and who knew the diagnosis of a team of doctors who had worked with Mother for over a year. The incident does point out that even in the *middle stages*, Alzheimer's disease is not always readily apparent even to trained medical professionals.

This Las Vegas trip was the beginning of major intervention by other family members. Until this time, Dad had been able to handle Mom on his own, with just a little support from family and friends when traveling.

Mother's medical care was through Group Health Cooperative, whom she had been with for years. Early in 1988 Group Health asked Mom and Dad if Mom would be willing to be part of a long-term Alzheimer's study being done at the University of Washington. This was something they both agreed to do, made even more interesting because Mom was still denying she had Alzheimer's. Mom went in for the first of the mental tests that spring. She came out of it severely depressed. She felt exposed, publicly humiliated. Dad said she cried and was upset over it for days. She said she would never do it again, and Dad said he would never let her do it again. Six months later it was time to go in again. Mother, believing in research and wanting to make a difference, willed herself to go. Again she came home emotionally ravished. Yet year after year when the time came to be re-tested, Mom went in and did it, and Dad supported her. Each time she was upset and depressed, and each time they agreed together to never do that again. Of course with every passing year, Mom knew less and less of what was going on. She went until she no longer knew what she was doing or where she was. It was the first I was to see of her great courage, and of Dad's too.

Mother struggled mightily during this period to retain the ability to think. Use of her mind was something she believed in to the core of her being. She still tried to read. She tried to do finances. She tried to keep up.

Meanwhile, I had been researching Alzheimer's, telling Dad I would keep him informed. Once Dad fairly hissed at me, "Are you sending literature to your mother about Alzheimer's? It is upsetting her terribly!" (In truth, his language was a bit more spicy than this, but that was the gist.) I hadn't sent anything to Mom. The Doctor herself was sending away for information. When it arrived, she had forgotten she had sent for it, and it reminded her of her ever-worsening mind.

In August of 1988 Dad and Homer hosted a reunion of all their Kansas school chums. Dad asked me to come up and help clean for the event. It wasn't difficult for me to do. Always generous, Dad had lent us his motor home for a family vacation, and we were on our way through Seattle to take it back anyway. When we got to their home it was obvious that Mom had been trying to get things ready. In my old bedroom, now a guest room, the bed was *mostly* made. There was a pile of sweepings on the hardwood floor, another unfinished task. Mother really had done quite a bit of work; she just needed someone to come along after her to finish things. The windows were another story. Once a master window washer, she was no longer able to do them at all. She would take her pan of water and vinegar and put it all over the windows and then walk away or just take a swipe at it and then leave! Homer said that at the reunion it was obvious to all that Mom's mind was going. The days of hiding the disease were now largely over.

Mom and Dad didn't lose their friends. It amazed all of us how close neighbors and friends stayed. Mom and Dad had belonged to a bridge club in their neighborhood for years. The bridge club stayed a close knit group throughout Mom's long illness. She continued to play right along with everyone else, even though her ability was surely affected. What good sports! There was a women's bridge club also in the neighborhood that Mom had belonged to off and on. The women in that club continued to call Mom to fill in for them long after it became obvious that her mind was slipping away. I gained such respect for Mom and Dad's friends throughout this period.

At Dad's request, I began to spread the word, though, that overnight company was becoming too burdensome for Mom and Dad. A few times it upset me that people ignored this, feeling that surely *they* were close enough to come for a visit. Surely *they* weren't a burden for Mom and Dad. By 1989, with Dad's health becoming precarious, too, there wasn't *anyone* who could come and not be a burden.

Dad was becoming the housekeeper now. He also undertook a project in their daylight basement. He built (with a little help from his friends . . .) a small apartment. He was thinking ahead, knowing the time for needing more help was coming soon.

Somewhere in this time frame, Mom and Dad took another trip to Alaska to visit Tom and Teri, even though traveling was becoming more difficult for Dad, too. On this trip Mom took little Jessie for a walk in the stroller and got lost. Fortunately, she was brought back home by a stranger, and Jessie was unharmed. Clearly, the Alzheimer's Mom was suffering from could also be dangerous. While she could still go on her daily walks at home, she could no longer go out alone away from familiar surroundings.

Ethical issues suddenly began to crop up all over the place. Of course it is important for Alzheimer's victims to maintain their independence for as long as possible. Certainly they resent any outside attempts to curtail it. But when do you begin to take these freedoms away? Dad felt so strongly that it was important to allow freedom and independence as long as possible . . . and maybe then some.

At one point Mom and Dad began getting overdue notices from the phone company. Dad asked Mom if she had paid the phone bill, and she assured him that she had. She had been paying the bills for years. Dad was kind of watching this, keeping loose track, as overdue notices cropped up from time to time. He knew also that she would pay for things twice and that she gave money to just about anyone who came to the door soliciting or selling. Although it was totally out of character for him, he just let these things go. But for some reason the phone company kept sending these notices, and this time it didn't stop. The phone service did stop, however, and Mom and Dad received a notice that their non-payment was going on their credit record. Dad of course instantly took care of the situation.

Then he did something truly amazing. Dad continued to allow Mother to pay the bills! Against everyone's advice, mine included, Dad kept his mailbox in front of the house rather than getting a post office box for business mail. "Your mother loves to get the mail. She goes to the mailbox about ten times a day!" He never said a word to her about the phone company again. He just simply began paying the bills *with* her. He began to stash the bills in a desk downstairs when she brought in the mail. When it was time to pay them, they did it together. Gradually, he was paying the bills alone, but by then she no longer noticed.

The car situation was pure poetry. Dad was an artisan when it came to handling people; he always had been. Handling someone with Alzheimer's was just a little trickier. When Mom got to the point where we wondered if she should drive, Dad never said a word. He never once told her she should not drive. He bought himself a truck. Mother hated it. A short time later, he sold her car! Now, Dad was a lifelong trader, a buyer and a seller. Mother had spent a lifetime putting up with a refrigerator that didn't match her kitchen because Dad had gotten a good deal on it. She settled for him selling things out from under her, so he could get something else. It was just his way. Having him sell her car was just another of his shenanigans, and she supposed she had to put up with it. She never drove after that.

Mother, until she lost the use of a car, was still shopping. Much like everything else in their lives, this took on a tinge of madness. Just as she asked the same questions again and again, mother seemed to get in a rut with shopping. She would buy the same items repeatedly. First it was chicken. She bought a few packages of chicken each week until the freezer was completely full of chicken. Then it was corn flakes. I don't think either of them ate corn flakes, but The Doctor bought them faster than Dad could give them away. When it came to toilet paper, Dad had had too much. Still, he said nothing to Mother. He merely called me long distance from a pay phone and wailed about toilet paper. Dad, who had never cared about the details of his life, who had a wife to take care of the mundane for him, Dad the great dreamer and wheeler dealer, and Dad the socialite, had been reduced to counting packages of toilet paper. That very morning he had counted no less than fifty-six packages of toilet paper in their house. "She has toilet paper everywhere! There is toilet paper on my workbench in the garage. There is toilet paper in the laundry room and broom closet. There is toilet paper in the kitchen and in our bedroom. There are 56 #@!*! packages of toilet paper in our !@#*! house!" I wasn't nearly as sympathetic as Dad needed at the time; I couldn't help laughing.

But not long after that, Mom had no car . . .

One of the things Dad said was, "If it never gets any worse than this, well then, we will be fine. We can handle this." I heard him say that many times for years. It was a beautiful expression of faith and optimism. It was his boundless "can-do" attitude.

Dad still traveled regularly, always with The Doctor in tow. Usually he took trips around the state. He went with Homer and Betty fishing at Conconully. He went clam-digging with us. Often a couple from the bridge club would travel with them. He no longer just went with Mom. He needed others to help—another woman to stop at public rest rooms or those in restaurants. Mother could go into a stall in a rest room and lock the door. Then she wouldn't know how to get out. If she did get out of the stall, she couldn't find her way out of the rest room. Or if she found her way out of the rest room, she couldn't find her way to the car. She might head in another direction. Dad was not in the good physical shape she was. She was hard to keep up with. These are just some examples of the problems of traveling with Mom. Dad worked hard at keeping his *life*. He fought its narrowing. He knew that the traveling was hard on Mom. She got so terribly confused. But it was a way for him to cope. It was something he needed to do for himself.

I returned to teaching in the fall of 1988, having been home raising children for fifteen years. By the spring of 1989 I was also commuting to Seattle, three hours each way, about once a month to check on Mom and Dad. I would do some cleaning, and usually I either cooked and put things away in the freezer (ready-to-eat meals), or I brought some meals that I had prepared at home. Dad wanted to go the TV dinner route, but I took him shopping and showed him how much sodium these meals had. His heart and blood pressure were troublesome, and he had diabetes, too. I got him into using a microwave. He was becoming the cook. John also came to check in on Mom and Dad from time to time. He lived several hours away by car but managed to get over several times a year. Tom in Anchorage was too far to come often, but he called Dad regularly and was a kindred spirit for Dad to talk to.

My Heather was about to become a senior in high school. One beautiful summer day I took her to meet a friend at the University of Washington for a look around. We took The Doctor with us, giving Dad a break. The girls went one way, while Mom and I had a leisurely walk and lunch. As we were talking about people from her bridge club, Mom said something about Stan Quande being 101 years old. Stan was around Mom's age (73) or younger, so he was nowhere near 101. I told Dad about it later, and he said that sometimes The Doctor would say something outrageous like that and then sometimes hear herself and realize that she sounded "like a damn fool." Of course she was embarrassed then. So neither Dad nor I corrected The Doctor when she said something we knew not to be true.

While it was important to listen to The Doctor, to hear her wants and needs, her information was not always reliable anymore. We had to be careful how we listened and weigh what she said.

At one time or another, Mom had seriously hurt the feelings of pretty much everyone she knew. I know for sure that she had hurt Auntie Ethel's feelings and Aunt Babe's. She had hurt her good friend Joan's feelings. Dad said she was rough on Homer and Betty as early as the Australia trip. The list went on and on. Auntie Ethel wondered once if Mother maybe just never did like her and now that her tact was gone, the truth was out? I assured her that Mother never had an unkind word about Auntie Ethel all the while I was growing up. I was sure these were not her true feelings. Early in the course of her Alzheimer's, The Doctor Agnes, K.E., had even managed to hurt the feelings of people who lived far away. One of Auntie Ethel and Uncle Harold's adult children had asked about coming to Seattle for a visit, and Mom had told them to stay away. This was totally out of character for her.

Near the end of 1989, as Mom's emotional problems increased, she also began sneaking up on Dad when he was relaxing in his chair in the living room. His recliner was next to the big picture window at the front of the house overlooking the water. With a quarter turn he could watch TV. Often he would doze off. The Doctor might get right behind him and then pull a single hair on the back of his head. I can imagine this did nothing to improve his heart condition! Mom would also sneak around to hear his phone conversations. He began to call me from other places when he wanted to talk. I think he did this with Homer, too. I asked Dad if he ever felt physically threatened by The Doctor. He said no, but she was right on the edge. It wasn't out of the realm of possibility. I told him if he ever did, he was to tell me, and I would take responsibility for her after that. He couldn't bear to think of her away from him.

Middle Dementia

Many changes occur during this stage of dementia. The Alzheimer's victim would not be able to survive alone at this stage. The role of the caregiver increases dramatically. Often the Alzheimer's patient requires full-time outside care either from a care facility or in the form of in-home care.

There are changes in this stage in personal hygiene, the ability to dress oneself, and sporadic episodes of incontinence. The ability to bathe or shower is impeded by the inability to adjust temperature of the water and the inability to get in and out of the bath, due to coordination problems.

Repetitive behaviors intensify. Once the person does the same thing at the same time more than once, chances are this will continue on a repetitive basis. Such behaviors may include leaving to go for a walk, shopping, taking things out of drawers, and many more.

Sleep disturbances occur at this stage. In fact, sleep disturbances are the most frequent reason for institutionalizing an Alzheimer's patient. It is difficult for a caregiver to be up night and day. For an Alzheimer's patient without medication, it is routine. Hallucinations, delusions, and paranoia increase. Fear becomes a part of the victim's life. It may be fear based on the loss of abilities. For example, it might be the fear of getting in the shower because of the inability to adjust the temperature. Perhaps it is related to the experience of having been burned or chilled. Fears may also appear that are not based in reality. These are paranoia. The caregiver is accused of unfaithfulness if it is a spouse, is accused of being an impostor, and so on. Violent behavior may occur at this stage. Agitation increases. It is difficult for the individual to rest. Coordination changes occur. This may manifest itself in a slower walk, problems with buttons and zippers, and so on. The loss of a sense of time and place also intensifies. Denial is no longer a useful coping mechanism. Verbal ability diminishes. The individual can no longer tell others what he or she needs (Gruetzner, 1988).

Chapter 7

1990

Mom and Dad headed for Las Vegas in January, stopping at our house on the way. Since it was Dad's 70th birthday, Ralph and I invited Homer and Betty down for a surprise. When Mom and Dad got here, they found Homer and Betty and a surprise party waiting for them.

After their trip, Dad found a couple to move into the basement apartment he had built. They were both mildly mentally handicapped. The young man was able to mow the lawn, do the gardening, and keep the place in repair. The young woman would sit with Mom, so Dad could get out during the day. She also did the laundry and some cleaning. In return, the couple got their little basement apartment and a small salary. The young man also had time to do handyman chores for others in the neighborhood who would hire him.

I sent a letter to a good friend in July of 1990. After describing the hectic spring we had at my house in Battle Ground with Heather's high school graduation, Janelle's confirmation, parades and concerts for Janelle, a play and many graduation activities for Heather, not to mention our jobs, I wrote this paragraph about Mom and Dad:

My folks are doing OK. Mom has finally admitted having a problem. It's depressing for her, but it would be for anyone. The burden is tough on Dad. He is so kind to her, it's amazing. He is becoming very domestic, fixing up the house, cooking, etc. He can't go like he used to either. I just hope his heart doesn't give out. It is a little stubbornness that keeps him going. He refuses to quit. They came down for graduation and confirmation. Mom and

*I somehow managed to gather up all four ducks (that I had raised
from ducklings) and move them to the creek. They had never been
farther than the back yard. And at dark Skipper (our dog) took it
upon himself to bring them back up! In the morning Mom and I
chased them back down, and that night Skipper brought them back
again. So now they come and sleep in the back yard every night
and at dawn they go quack-quacking back down to the creek—
which is probably safer for them anyway.*

Obviously, The Doctor was in very good shape physically. She still walked
to the beach every day from her home. My parents' neighborhood owned
a stretch of beach on Puget Sound. It was a little community beach, a
wonderful retreat from the city. It was perhaps a half mile walk each way,
and usually The Doctor walked on the beach before the steep climb home.
This was a walk she had been doing for nearly thirty years, and she never
got lost on it. Of course, everyone along the way knew her.

On one of my weekend voyages to Seattle, I walked with Mom down
to the beach. It was just after a rain, and the rocks were slippery. The tide
was out, and so we went beach combing. The Doctor Agnes, K.E., liked
pretty rocks especially, while I was partial to shells and—my real weak-
ness—driftwood. Mother often brought things up from the beach. It was not
uncommon for her to come home with her pockets full of treasures. Her
patio was strewn with shells, driftwood, and rocks. Then she also had
mounted rocks on driftwood and hung it on the side of her house like a
picture. When we headed back that cloudy day, not thinking, I led her over
the big rocks up to the picnic area where our path home began. We could
have gone around a longer way, but Mom and I were used to climbing over
the boulders that lined the bulkhead. Mom slipped that day, and I watched
in horror as her head went down in a kind of slow motion. She looked like
a doll falling with no reflex. She wasn't knocked out, thank Heaven, but
she had hit her head and the side of her face quite hard. Her hands had not
gone down to break her fall. I made her sit for half an hour or so to make
sure she was all right before we headed home. I didn't want her walking up
the steep hill if she had a concussion. She kept saying how lucky she was
that she didn't break anything. It was typical of her outlook on life. I didn't

think she looked very lucky with her face all bruised, but she was grateful that it hadn't been worse! Later I told Ralph that I had never understood how older people could hurt themselves so badly in a fall. Now, after seeing Mom and the absolute absence of her reflexes, I could understand it.

Mom's clothing began to look shabby during this period. I am sure shopping in a mall by herself was out of the question. I don't think she ever thought to shop. When Betty or Auntie Ethel or I would mention this to Dad, he became both hurt and outraged. He was sure she had plenty of clothes. Actually, she did. They were all just old. But she looked beautiful to him. He really didn't think to get her any either. I began to buy Mom clothes for her birthdays and other occasions. Others did, too. Still, she was partial to her familiar old things, and so she looked less well-kept than she could have. Betty began taking Mom to have her hair done. Dad was doing the best that he could, so this was probably the least of his worries. Perspective.

Dad was finding that he had to take Mom's clothes out of their room to wash them or else she would keep wearing the same thing day after day. Auntie Ethel did this for them when they were in Las Vegas.

Inevitably, Dad's life was narrowing. His arteries were clogging up again, so his own health was worsening. He had to do more and more at home to keep things going there. Mother was continually more difficult to manage.

Once I took Mom to the mall and told Dad I was going to spend some money. As mentioned before, aluminum has been a suspect in causes of Alzheimer's, and much of Mom's old cookware was bare aluminum. Even though this was a classic case of "closing the barn door after the cows had gotten out," I felt Mom really didn't need any more aluminum. So we went out and bought some new cookware, and I charged it on one of Mom's credit cards. (She always had to have her purse, and Dad had not taken a thing out of it. By this time it carried everything from curlers to playing cards to scotch tape, but I managed to find a wallet in there, too.) I also got her a new outfit.

By now, Mom's drawers and cupboards were looking much like the inside of her purse. It was very difficult to find things. I began trying to clean the kitchen cupboards when I came. I even offered to label the cupboards, but Dad said he thought it was too late for that. He was probably right. Still, it might have helped earlier.

There were many niggling problems Dad was facing with Mom. She would leave on burners on the stove, for example. She caused a couple of small fires in 1990. Dad and I talked about re-wiring the stove, putting a switch in the cupboard below. Dad was thinking about future care for Mom as his own health declined.

When Dad quit drinking years before, he had done it on his own, "cold turkey." No AA for him. He was never the support-group type. Of course many people had told him that there were support groups for caregivers of Alzheimer's victims. Never did anyone dream that *he* would take advantage of them. Everyone was surprised when Dad started going to these meetings. He made friends there, as he did everywhere. Most importantly, he learned things. He learned to take the knobs off the stove and put them in a drawer. Mom couldn't get through the process of wanting to use the stove, looking for the knobs, finding the knobs and putting them on, and remembering what she was doing at the stove. Just putting the knobs in the silverware drawer stopped the fires. Dad also learned about foster care for the elderly at his support group meetings. He went with one man to visit his wife in a foster care home. Of course Dad wasn't ready for that yet. "If it never gets any worse than this, we'll be fine."

By the end of 1990, Mom was into taking things out of drawers and closets, packing suitcases, and telling Dad that she wanted to go home. This was happening *at home*. It was another example of losing perspective of time and place, and an example of repetitious behavior, but it made Dad feel guilty for traveling all the time. He felt as if she was haunted by it. Certainly he was. In truth, this is common behavior for an Alzheimer's patient in the middle dementia stage.

Another of the Doctor's repetitive habits centered on bananas and ice-cream. Dad generally had ice cream in the freezer for her, and she would help herself, sometimes several times a day. She did the same thing with bananas. Then Dad would fix them a meal, and she wouldn't be able to eat much. "Too full." Somehow her weight remained about the same throughout her bananas and ice cream phase.

Christmas of 1989 had been very hard on Mom and Dad, even though Denise, Teri, and I had done most of the cooking. Overnight company— even family—was rough. Dad still insisted on having Christmas at their house the next year. We decided that for Christmas of 1990 we would again have it at their house. Tom, Teri, and Jessie were even coming down from Alaska. I think Dad knew it would be his last Christmas. His heart condition was considered inoperable. Mom was not able to do anything for Christmas. Teri, Denise, and I were to make the meal. So we divvied up the tasks and had Christmas dinner. Dad was short-tempered with John. Tom and Teri's last visit with the folks in Alaska had been very strained. Everyone was a little stressed, but we got through it, and then Mom began to cry as we were cleaning up afterwards. I asked her why she was crying, and she said that Christmas had come and gone in her own house but that she wasn't even part of it anymore. I put my arms around her and apologized for making the dinner. I told her that we had wanted it to be a treat for her. Teri, Denise, and I had made the dinner as a Christmas gift to her; we hadn't done it to exclude her. She stopped crying then and let us clean up, with her "helping." In all honesty, Mom was hardly able to boil water at this point.

Chapter 8

1991

Mom and Dad waited until after the first of the year to venture down to Las Vegas. This time Dad couldn't make the trip down without help for Mom. Long time family friends Eleanor Williams and Ruth Arnold were also heading south. They came along with Mom and Dad for the trip. Eleanor and Ruth were both widows now, but a more fun duo would be difficult to find. Since Dad's 71st birthday was in January, we celebrated that when the four of them stopped for an overnight on their way. Dad looked so cute. He had a new leather jacket and a sporty cap. He looked like the cat that ate the canary, taking three women to Vegas!

Mom and Dad also went down to El Paso again, even though Dad's health wasn't too great. Aunt Babe called just after they had left her place, and she told me that Dad had a bad chest cold and did not look good when they left. Back in Las Vegas, Dad's "chest cold" got so bad that Auntie Ethel put him—forcibly—in the hospital. He had pneumonia and congestive heart failure again, and his kidneys began to shut down also. He was truly rescued from the jaws of death this time. The doctor told him when he began to recover that if he had come in even a few hours later, it would have been all over.

Again John flew down to Las Vegas to bring them home. This time Auntie Ethel and Uncle Harold followed John back up in their motor home and stayed to care for Dad and Mom for a short time. Uncle Harold had been battling cancer, so this gift of time from them was an act of pure self-lessness. Harold and Dad had a bet going on who would enter the Pearly Gates first. I'm not sure how they decided the "loser" would pay up.

I began a weekly commute to Seattle on the weekends to cook and shop. It was becoming obvious that the young couple caring for Dad and The Doctor were in over their heads. I had been researching retirement and nursing homes in my area while Mom and Dad were in Vegas. I began to urge Dad to consider coming down to the Vancouver area.

By Easter, Dad was feeling better. He and Mom met us halfway between Seattle and Vancouver for Easter dinner. He looked good, but Ralph noticed some incontinence then, that Dad was "leaking" just a little.

That spring, Mom was having serious emotional problems. Once she went downstairs to the little apartment and began screaming and crying that Dad was cheating on her with the young woman who was helping. She cried often. I would try to talk to her by phone, and she would just begin to cry. There was no way to reason with her.

Then Mom got the flu and was deathly ill for over a month. She had always been a good sleeper. But often in 1991 she would not sleep at night. She was given some medication to help with sleep and with her emotions. When she got the flu she just slept and slept. This was what Mom had always done on the rare occasions of her life when she got sick. Now it gave Dad a rest.

In May, Dad began to have some kidney pain. He went to the doctor and found that he had a kidney stone. He was definitely not a good candidate for surgery, so an attempt was made to treat it with drugs, hoping to dissolve the stone. Dad went out and bought a Lincoln Towne Car, brand new, undoubtedly to lift his spirits. Eleanor Williams, who had been to Las Vegas with them, kindly offered to help him take care of it . . .

Dad's doctors were also telling him that he could no longer care for Mom. They told him to put her in a nursing home, that within a few days she would be "banging on pots and not know the difference." They were wrong on two counts. First, she would know the difference. Second, the move would not save Dad; it would kill him. Fortunately, Dad knew that he couldn't do it anyway. His doctors were correct that things needed to change, that Dad could no longer take care of Mom alone.

Dad, Homer, and I got together to decide what to do for Mom's care. In truth, of course, Dad needed care, too. Suggesting professional live-in care, I found a woman named Sandy who had excellent references and would be available soon. I set up an appointment for her to meet Dad and

Homer for an interview later that week. Sandy looked like a very good alternative, so she was hired, and the young couple was given plenty of notice and references and let go.

It was finally decided that Dad was going to have surgery for the kidney stone. My school was out, so I took care of Mother during the surgery. John also spent quite a bit of time with Dad in the hospital. Shortly after the surgery, Dad suffered a minor heart attack.

When Dad got out of the hospital, Aunt Babe and Uncle Larry were visiting from Texas. They stayed just a few days, and Dad said later that he thought he had another small heart attack at that time. Babe and Larry dropped Mom off at my house on their way back to Texas, and Sandy was installed to take care of Dad at home in Seattle. Sandy had been told that the closets and cupboards were all a mess, thanks to The Doctor's busyness. Sandy set to work right away cleaning that up and washing all of Mom's clothes and linens.

Back at my house Mother was indeed a full-time job. She had to be watched constantly. Our home was located in the middle of a forest, and if she got lost around my house she could be lost in the woods for days without ever seeing anyone. That was a worry.

The Doctor Agnes, K.E., liked to pick blackberries at the edge of the woods around our house. She enjoyed going with me on walks up the hill. She liked the dog and cats, the birds and other small wildlife. She liked being a part of life. I took Janelle and some friends to the ocean for a day with The Doctor in tow. She had a wonderful day, and I bought her a new pink sweatshirt for her birthday, since pink was what she wanted to wear.

The Doctor had to be helped to bathe by this time. I ran a bath for her and helped her undress and get in. Then I let her to soak for a while before coming back to wash her face and back. I washed her hair at the kitchen sink. She could get dressed, but I had to put out clean clothes for her each day and take dirty ones away. And of course she was so messy! By the time the summer was over, all of my drawers had been "rearranged."

The worst of caring for The Doctor was at night. We had to keep the doors locked at night and the keys kept out of sight for fear that she would get out. Since the bedrooms are upstairs, we kept the lights on in the hall-ways and put up a guardrail used for babies, so she wouldn't fall down the stairs. Then there were the times we would wake up in the middle of the night and Mother would be standing in our room smiling at us. It was one step beyond weird. When we built our home, our girls had wanted locks on their bedroom doors. We put them on, but Heather and Janelle were told, for fire safety, never to lock their doors at night. Both girls had "visitations" from Mom at night before Ralph and I did. Once we had been "visited," I told them to lock their doors at night. Their granny also tried to crawl into bed with them.

Ralph was my rock during this time. He was (and is) just steady. While I am emotional, a bit of a dreamer, and I tend to operate in either high gear or low, Ralph lives at a steady, even pace. I never had to ask if he minded me running back and forth to Seattle; he just took care of things at home, so I could go. He never made a single negative comment about The Doctor being with us over the summer. When I tried to draw Ralph out, tried to get him to express his feelings, he said he felt "inadequate to do anything" to help Mom, something I found surprising since I felt he had helped so much. But he meant that he couldn't make her better. He also admitted that he felt increasingly "repelled ... but not revolted" by her, even though he had always been fond of his mother-in-law. His honesty helped me to understand others whose reactions were different from my own.

It was hard on Janelle and Heather to share me. Heather never complained directly. She was just generally miffed that I had not taken the time to come to visit her at college in Salem more often during the school year and to get to know her new college friends. I had a hard time relating to Heather's complaints since Dad and Mom had *never* visited me in college— and I lived in the same town! From my perspective, visiting Heather a few times each year, plus having her home once or twice a semester seemed about right. But she felt differently, and that was her right. In the summer my involvement with The Doctor didn't make much difference to her. Heather was good at handling her. She would sit at the piano and play old hymns and generally enjoyed helping with her.

Janelle had a harder time being around a demented person. It upset her. It also angered her that I was having to spend so much time with Mom and Dad. Mom and Dad had been jet-setters, to be sure. They spent a great deal of time with friends and neighbors. They had no time for us until the

Alzheimer's became a problem. In our Spokane neighborhood, Janelle had a "pretend grandmother," Mrs. Eymer. Mrs. Eymer bought her a gift on her birthday. Mrs. Eymer sent her a postcard when she went on trips. Mrs. Eymer brought her souvenirs of shells and necklaces. Mrs. Eymer was someone who gave her cookies and Coke after school and listened to her trials and triumphs. Mrs. Eymer died suddenly at the end of 1990. And Janelle was not done grieving Mrs. Eymer. Furthermore, Janelle had Mrs. Eymer to contrast with her "real" grandparents, who had never remembered birthdays or sent postcards from their trips. More than once we had traveled hundreds of miles to visit, only to have Mom and Dad *leave* the minute we got there! Dad might need to go talk business to someone, while Mom ran off to play bridge. Janelle could remember our first Christmas in Battle Ground when we planned to have Christmas dinner with my folks. Three days before Christmas they called to wonder if we'd mind if they had Christmas dinner with some friends from Kansas who were in town. We weren't invited. This was, of course, just the tip of a rather large iceberg. Janelle was no fool. By the summer of 1991 and 15 years old, she told me point blank, "I just don't have any respect for people who don't have time for me until they need me." She felt we were being used. It was a point I never tried to argue.

I was keenly aware, however, that I had two daughters watching how I cared for my aging parents. I wanted them to take note of it, whether they liked it or not. Parents are first and foremost models for their children. I had a vested interest in setting a good example here; the day could come when *I* might need help from my children. The point I did tell my children was the Golden Rule. "Do unto others as you would have others do unto you." We are not called to treat people the way we feel like treating them. Nor are we called to treat others the way they have treated us. We are called to treat them the way *we* would *like* to be treated. I personally had struggled with this even before the beginning of Mother's Alzheimer's. I became first convinced of it, then committed to it, and finally freed by it. Freed of needing to judge and weigh how I had been treated. Free of weighing my response to it. Free of guilt. Just committed and free. It was the narrow door that enabled me to lose my own hang-ups and take care of the business at hand. This did not occur overnight. It would be hard to say that it was an actual event or a single choice. It was more a spiritual and emotional process, a walk that happened over time. I knew that I had to empty myself, to let go of my own feelings to do this. There were and would be many times when I would feel the old hurts or be haunted by memories. Yet a conscious choice was made to not let the past poison my present and future. We had a pastor who was fond of saying in his sermons, "You can't drive forward by looking in your rear-view mirror." By the summer of 1991, with both Dad and The Doctor considerably incapacitated, I was sure and firm on the course I had chosen and committed to, and I was able to articulate it to Heather and Janelle, so they could understand.

I also felt that taking care of older parents is a natural part of life. Each stage of life, regardless of how difficult, is meaningful, valuable, and worthwhile. I did not want to be denied this in my life for any reason.

What I didn't know in 1991 was that as my "self" was shed over the years and the drudgery gave way to routine, there would be joy, new memories, and new friends. We would have some fun. The journey would engage my intellect, imagination, and heart. I didn't know then that the trip would be so worth taking. I only knew it was one that I somehow needed to take.

It is never easy to balance having a full-time job and children at home. That was the reason I stayed home for fifteen years. It is even more difficult doing this and taking care of aging parents. I had just started back to work as a teacher and hadn't even adjusted to that, when care for Mom and Dad became an issue. I was feeling fully the effects of being in the sandwich generation. Many times choices were made about time with Heather, Janelle, and Ralph or time with Mom and Dad. Although it may look as Mom and Dad always won out, that being the subject of this book, it was not always the case. Ralph and I enjoyed taking a day off to spend with Heather installing her in her dorm at school in the fall, helping her set up a checking account, taking her for lunch. We went to parents' weekend at Willamette University. We each took time to go down and take her out for lunch or dinner. We never missed a concert for Janelle or a play for either of the girls. They both had free use of the house for their own parties and entertainment; we were there for all of these. Until they could drive they were both transported to lessons, activities, and the homes of friends, necessary because of our home in the country. Ralph and I had committed to the transportation because we didn't want our girls to pay a price just because their parents wanted to live in the country. I was stretched pretty thin, but I was also guilt-free.

Around the end of July we took Mom to John and Denise in Idaho, so we could have a little vacation visiting friends across the border in Spokane, and so I could have some time off before school started. It felt so *freeing* to be out from under the responsibility for a while. John and Denise were to take care of Mom for a few weeks and then take her to Seattle, where theoretically, Dad would be better, and he and Sandy would take it from there.

John and Denise's children, Andrew and Natalie, were also in for some upset. Living with Mom was like living with Goldilocks; she had to try every bed! They did not know what to make of their grandmother coming and moving everything around. Andrew lost a wallet and was sure Granny had taken it—which she had. It was upsetting and hard for these elementary-school-age children to understand why Granny would steal from them. Natalie and Andrew had been quite close to their grandparents. Denise's family lived near their house in Seattle, so there had been quite a bit of interaction. After a couple of weeks in Idaho, The Doctor returned to her home in Seattle, to the relief of all.

We now all understood how hard Dad had been working to take care of The Doctor. None of us had fully realized the extent of Mom's craziness until then, or the extent of her inability for her to care for herself. Actually having to take care of her ourselves was an eye-opener.

Meanwhile, Dad was having problems getting along with Sandy. Truthfully, Dad was having problems getting along with anyone. He was mad at Mom's pastor for not sending people to take Mom to church. He had called the man and cussed him out! He'd upset Tom and Teri in Anchorage; he'd upset John at Christmas; he was mad at Homer and me for telling him to try to get along with Sandy. Sandy was a good cook and a good housekeeper. She did well with The Doctor, and she was dependable. She completely took over. Dad thought she spent too much money for groceries. Dad was just not feeling good. He was, in fact, dying. And he wasn't happy about it. First and foremost he didn't know what was going to happen to The Doctor.

I had found a retirement apartment in Vancouver, Washington, not far from my job with an assisted living wing for when The Doctor got worse. Homer drove Dad to Vancouver in the new Lincoln Towne Car, and I met them at the Cascade Inn. The administrator, Connie Easter, interviewed them to make sure they would be a good fit. Connie was trying to balance providing a retirement apartment for healthy retirees with the growing need to address Alzheimer's victims. She had told me she might be willing to admit Mom and Dad, but she wanted a look at them first.

After Connie met Mom and Dad, she told them she had a few questions for The Doctor. Her first was, "Who is the president?" Mom thought about this and said that Dad was and looked at Dad and me for confirmation. Both Dad and I had also taken Connie's question to mean, "Who is the boss in this relationship?" We both looked back at Mom and said, "Yes, Dad is the president." Connie probably thought "This whole family is loony tunes," but she graciously said, with a smile, "Who is the president of the United States?" Of course Mom had no idea. Connie asked her to name any president, and this Mom could not do either. She just said, "I don't know." Then Connie said, "Which of these was a president: Walter Cronkite, Richard Nixon, or Tom Jones?" Mother raised her hand and nodded when Connie said "Richard Nixon." Dad was so brave during that meeting. Not feeling well, he was brave to even make the trip down. Connie showed them a two-bedroom apartment that was available, and they took it.

Dad had been telling me, John, and Tom for several months to decide which of their things each of us wanted when he was gone. Like The Doctor Agnes, K.E., he didn't want us fighting about anything afterwards. We all said that we couldn't think of a thing, but it was a good idea on his part to get us thinking about it. He'd gotten his financial affairs all in order over the past few years, liquidating and consolidating. He had consulted with an attorney and a financial planner and gotten control of financial matters legally removed from Mother. He had set up his will so that assets were divided between his wife and children. He took on the work of this planning as soon as The Doctor had been diagnosed with Alzheimer's. John and I had been shown where everything was, and he had gone over his will with us.

August 15th was Sandy's last day. Friends came to help Dad with Mom for a couple of days. I was scheduled to go to Seattle on the 18th, there to meet Tom, John, Homer and Betty for the move. I decided to go on the 17th instead. When I got there Dad said to me, "I had been *praying* you would come today." It was quite an admission for Dad, and I knew he wasn't feeling well.

On the 18th I said to Dad after breakfast, "I want you to sit in your chair, and I don't want you to get out of it until we are all packed up. Then you can have a walk around the house and tell us if there is anything we've forgotten." He agreed, but being the consummate sidewalk supervisor, I knew he'd never do it. Tom arrived from Anchorage and John from Idaho. Homer and Betty came, and the move was on. I felt so guilty moving Mom and Dad out of their home of thirty years. I knew *I* wouldn't want to be treated like that; I was breaking the Golden Rule. I'll never forget the feeling.

We were about three quarters of the way finished with loading up when Mom began to notice things were not the way they had been. She just began to get nervous, pacing, wild-eyed, and agitated. Betty suggested a walk to the beach.

When they got back, there were just some big pieces of furniture left to be loaded. I looked at Dad—who had not moved from his chair since morning—and said, "It's time for you to look through the house now." So he did.

Mom, Dad, and I drove to my house outside Battle Ground while the others finished loading. Mom and Dad had a rest there while Ralph, John, and Tom unloaded at the Cascade Inn in nearby Vancouver. They then came back to Battle Ground for dinner. Afterwards I took Mom and Dad to their new home. Their beds had been made up. I told Dad I'd be back the next day to hang pictures and finish the unpacking.

Their first week at the Cascade Inn, Mom and Dad just rested. Dad said he slept the whole time, and Mom seemed content just to sit near him. They only left the apartment for meals in the dining room, although they had a kitchenette in their apartment. Housekeeping services were provided there, as was entertainment, church services, postal services, and transportation for outings. Nevertheless, they brought the new Lincoln Towne Car, which had covered parking.

One day I came to have lunch with them. Dad said to me, "Your mother is the best looking woman in this place." I kind of started to laugh, and he was outraged! "Well, just look around! She is!" Of course the place was full of women. Men were outnumbered by about eight-to-one. Dad had checked out all the women and decided he had the best of the bunch.

Connie also arranged to let Dad take The Doctor over to the Assisted Living Wing for a while on some days, so he could go out and play poker. He managed to do just that a couple of times and enjoyed a couple of the activities at the Cascade Inn. Ralph had told Dad to call him if he needed any little thing, and so he did some errands for Dad and helped him get settled, too.

Not long after they moved in, Mom got out of their apartment in just her underwear. So after that, each night before they went to bed, Dad had The Doctor move the kitchen table in front of their door, so she couldn't get out. Each night Mother wondered why she was moving the table!

My school started, and it looked as if Mom and Dad were finally settled nearby. The Cascade Inn was very near my school. I was grateful for a year where I wouldn't be running to Seattle every time I turned around.

Then Dad got a chest cold. He called at 4:00 A.M. one morning saying that he couldn't sleep; he couldn't stop coughing. He was short of breath. Arriving by 4:30, we had him in the hospital by 4:45. I didn't think that he was too bad, but they did blood gas tests on him in the Emergency Room and then admitted him.

I got the day off and took Mom back to the Inn, where Connie made arrangements with Assisted Living to have Mother each day from 8:00 A.M. until 4:00 P.M. It was a stretch for the Assisted Living Wing to do this, as they were set up with activities from 10:00 A.M. until 3:00 P.M. Connie arranged for the extra time, though. Each day between activities, The Doctor would walk in the halls and ask those who passed by, "Where's Charlie?"

Back at the hospital I met the cardiologist. Dad gave him some of his history. When he got to the part where he took three women to Las Vegas in January, Dr. Lavelle threw up his hands and exclaimed, "Well anyone who takes three women to Las Vegas is *asking* for heart failure!" Dad liked Dr. Lavelle right away, but that didn't change the diagnosis—another case of congestive heart failure.

After school each day, I took Mom to the hospital to visit Dad. Then we went to my home and had dinner. I gave her a bath, put her to bed, finished my school work, goofed off with Janelle, and called it a day. Janelle and Ralph were doing all the cooking and errands for a time.

Dad had been assigned another doctor, Dr. Manuela Laderas, an internist. Even though she was very thorough, she was a woman and Dad would have preferred a man. Dad had a couple of minor infections that she treated right away. Dr. Laderas called me on the phone and asked many questions in an effort to get a sense of this person, the patient. What had been his occupation? His hobbies? Was Mother his first and only wife? She wanted to know it all. Dr. Laderas never suggested to Dad that he should live apart from Mom. She did tell him that he might have to be in a nursing home or maybe a wheel chair for a while when he left the hospital.

Initially, it looked as if Dad might come around. His first few days brought steady improvement. Then he had another minor heart attack. When he first entered the hospital, he had signed a DNR (Do Not Resuscitate order). This instructed staff that he didn't want to be revived should he have a massive attack. Now he thought maybe he shouldn't have that. Dr. Lavelle had a talk with him, and he told Dad that it was, of course, his choice. He also said that if he should suffer a major attack at this point, his heart was so damaged that he would surely end his days as a "vegetable." That may not have been Dr. Lavelle's exact word, but it was the idea. Dad decided to leave the DNR in place. I later thanked Dr. Lavelle for his wise and difficult counsel.

Nevertheless, each shift of nurses asked *me* about the DNR. Was it really what I wanted? Of course hospitals have to "cover their fannies." Many states have regulations putting this responsibility into the relatives' hands. But I wasn't expecting this, maybe because Dad was so obviously coherent. I sensed that if I—or any other family member—hesitated on this question, Dad would indeed be resuscitated if he went into cardiac arrest. I answered carefully, "That really isn't the question, whether *I* want a DNR order on Dad. The question is, 'Will I honor *his* request for a DNR order?'

And my answer is that I will." This satisfied them, and it relieved me of a heavy responsibility.

Dad told me that he didn't want to exist as a "vegetable." "Pull the plug. Don't let them keep me that way." Then he said the same was to be for Mom. "Don't let anyone just keep her alive!" He was very emotional about this. I assured him that I wouldn't allow anyone to artificially maintain their lives. I'd let them go naturally when their time came. But Dad persisted. "They'll do it anyway, Charlotte!" Finally I looked at him and said evenly, "Now, Dad, you *know* me. You *know* what a big stink I can make if I'm unhappy. Do you honestly believe that I won't be able to have my way on this?" A slow little smile of peace came upon his face. He relaxed. "No, I'm sure you'll have your way," he said.

Dad wanted to see John. Because Tom in Alaska was so much farther away, John had only been bouncing across the countryside on a fairly constant basis for the last year helping Dad. John asked me on the phone if I really thought it was necessary that he come this time, too. It had been only a month since John and Tom had helped move The Doctor and Dad to Vancouver. It was an awful position to put me in, and I told him so. In the strictest sense it was not *necessary* that he come. Things were in hand. I said that I thought that it was *important* that he come. So he came.

Tom called from Anchorage wondering if he should come. John told him no, he had seen Dad look worse, particularly last winter in Vegas. Probably Dad would be getting to go home in a few days.

The next day, Dad had another small heart attack. The day after, when I brought Mom to visit, she was all flushed and pretty. She had her hair done that day at the Cascade Inn. There had been square dancing with a live band and she had "danced up a storm!" Then she looked at her poor husband in a hospital bed, felt a little guilty, and blushed some more. Dad giggled at her. He was so pleased to see her happy and having fun.

That night I called my sister Mary Lou's son, John, and told him that his Grandpa wasn't doing well. I called other relatives, as well as Homer and Betty. I called Heather at college, Auntie Ethel, Aunt Babe, and the Battle Ground pastor and bridge partner that Dad liked. Dad had once told me this pastor, Reverend Paul Tuchardt, was "the man for the job if you really need someone to grumble over my bones."

Dad wasn't doing very well the next day. He asked me not to bring Mom when I came. John and I stayed at the hospital for a while. Pastor had been there. Mary Lou's son, John, came, and we visited for an hour or so. John (Leonard) and I left to go to my house for dinner and to put The Doctor to bed. Then we went back to the hospital. I asked John to stop and buy me a pack of cigarettes. He said, "I didn't know you smoked!" I said, "I don't" and lit a cigarette as we drove on.

When we got to Dad's room, there were three nurses around him trying to get a pulse. Dad was fully conscious and coherent; he asked them to leave. They didn't. So he asked the nurses again. When he started to ask the third time, John told them to get the hell out of there. Then Dad tried to sit up. He said he wanted to talk to us. He convulsed and fell forward. And he was gone.

John left the room, but I needed to stay until his body was still. A nurse tried to tell me that Dr. Laderas was on the phone. I told her the doctor could call back. When a soul departs this earth it is time for a prayer, not a phone conversation. When it was over, a nurse asked if we wanted to donate his eyes. Of course we said, "Yes." Dad had such wonderful vision. Just yesterday he had read the stock market prices to me out loud from the newspaper. He wasn't even wearing his glasses. I also told the nurse that Mother had to come to visit first.

Another of The Doctor's lectures when she worked at Yarrington's Funeral Home was about the importance of the next of kin viewing the body. This, she explained more than any of us wanted to know, was so that the reality of it would sink in. It seemed to help those grieving.

The first thing I did was to call Ralph and tell him to get Mom to the hospital ASAP. When she came, I showed her that Dad had died. She patted on him, kissed him, cried, and told him how she had loved him so. For a moment, she was completely herself and whole and with us.

After that, the searching for Dad stopped, although she would still ask for him.

John went to Seattle to begin funeral arrangements. I moved Mom out of her retirement apartment the next day and into a little room in the Assisted Living Wing. I couldn't deal with her at home and arrange a funeral at the same time. In just over a month she had gone from living in a large home overlooking Puget Sound to living in a small room with a single bed, her desk, and chest of drawers. I felt guilty again.

When Mom and Dad first moved to the Cascade Inn, I had ordered an identification bracelet for Mom. The Inn was near a busy street. It had a shopping center to the east of it and a regular neighborhood with some duplexes, homes, and apartments to the west. The worry from the start was that The Doctor would get "loose." She had never stayed all night at the Inn without Dad. She had always come home with me or been with him. After tucking her into bed, I checked their mailbox one last time, hoping for the bracelet. There it was! I felt like my guardian angel—or hers!—had put it there just in time. I went back to her room and put it around her wrist. She was asleep already.

Four days later we took Mom to Seattle for the funeral. She really didn't understand all of what was going on. I had an insert made for the funeral program with Mom's new phone number and address, as well as a little map of how to get to her place. Many of her friends headed south in the winter. I wanted them to be able to find her if they were so inclined.

After the funeral we had a party back at her house. She'd had many parties there just like it. She looked beautiful in her pink dress. She sat among friends and visited. I doubt if it ever occurred to her that it was her husband's funeral. It was just as well that she couldn't comprehend the magnitude of her losses that beautiful fall day.

When she left, it was the last time she would ever see her home.

Ralph took Mom back home to the Cascade Inn, and I spent the night at Ruthie Arnold's house in Seattle. I met with Tom and John the next day, and we decided who would get what and how we were going to divide what needed to be done.

Tom was put in charge of the house. He was to do the cleanup and garage sale. Basically he was to get the house ready to rent or sell. We also told Tom to have Mary Lou come over if she wanted to, so that she could go through the things and take whatever she wanted.

John was put in charge of the finances. He was to work with the attorney on the will, decide how to invest any money, and pay Mother's bills. Dad had divided his will in half. Half was to go to Mom, the other half to be divided among his heirs. He did this so that we would get something in case Mom's care turned out to be so expensive that it used up his entire estate. He reasoned that she could go on Medicaid. We talked about this at length and decided that if we left the estate together, Mom might be able to live on the interest, her Social Security, and any income from the house's rental or sale. If we divided it in half, she would probably use half of it up fairly quickly. By leaving it together, we would end up with all or nearly all the estate upon Mom's death. We could also assure her of better care. If at any point it wasn't working, if the cost of her care was eroding the whole estate, we could execute the will right away, dividing it as Dad had. We Leonard "kids" were pretty sharp. We also decided that the money in the estate for our two older aunts should be offered to them right away; we could easily settle that part now, since they weren't getting any younger, and the money might afford them a trip or something they needed now.

I was put in charge of Mother, being responsible for her care. I was to set up a checking account for her, with my name on it as well, for her Social Security checks to be deposited. This turned out to be a far easier way to handle Social Security than trying to go through all the paperwork of them releasing the checks to me because she was mentally incompetent. We simply had the Social Security checks direct deposited in her account and since along with her name, my name and Ralph's were on the account, we could handle things for her. Of course it took me a month and many phone calls to figure this out. The bank helped me infinitely more than the Social Security office did.

Mom would have been proud of how well we got along handling Dad's and her affairs. We managed to get through it all without so much as a cross word between us!

Inevitably, there were changes in The Doctor over the course of Dad's decline. The worsening emotional problems, sleep disorders, and repetitious removal of things from drawers were all part of the process. Dad told me that the fears Mom had that spring were the worst of the Alzheimer's.

She would wake up terrified in the night, sometimes screaming or crying. She had a new medication, desipramine, that helped this finally.

There was another shift, too. When Auntie Ethel and Uncle Harold helped John bring Mom and Dad home from Vegas, Mom was pretty nasty to everyone. She was angry and accusing. She fought their help. By the summer, when Mother stayed with me, she was compliant and sweet. There had been a definite change of mood in her. The terrible fears were over.

Dad did us an enormous favor by hanging on as long as he did. Had he died while Mom was still regularly wandering or before Mom became docile, she may have ended up immediately restrained in a nursing home. Dad did not let go until he saw Mom happy and well cared for—without him. After the square dance, he was satisfied. I had told him that I would take care of Mother, that he need not worry. He needed to see for himself that she could go on without him. He also did both The Doctor and me a favor by moving her down near me before he died. Afterwards, I could say to Mother, to help orient her and to calm her, "Dad moved down here with you." Sometimes she would faintly remember.

Another change in The Doctor began in the spring of 1991. I came to think of it as "The Journey Back." This was the most intellectually fascinating part of Alzheimer's for me. Mom fixated on a period of her life when she and Dad were first married. They were living in Oregon, and she was the assistant or secretary to the president of a university. This university president made a pass at her, which shocked and outraged her. Nobody, including Dad, knew anything about it until the spring of 1991 when Mom relived that period over and over again. By that time, of course, Dad found it amusing. But Mom was shocked and outraged afresh almost daily for a while. The thing that made this so interesting was that Mother took on the mannerisms and thinking of a young woman. It wasn't that she was dwelling *on* the past. She was dwelling *in* it.

When Dad was in the hospital dying, Mom was then young and single. She blushed easily, flirted with a young man who was an assistant director of the Cascade Inn, and wanted to go to dances and parties. This is what Dad was seeing when she came and confessed that she had been dancing all day. He saw the young woman he had fallen in love with.

For the remainder of Mom's life, she journeyed back.

Without Dad, away from her home, her mind mostly gone, The Doctor was truly "lost in space." The extent of her helplessness terrified me. Stopping at the Cascade Inn, often before and after school, I put her clothes back in drawers, took her laundry home, walked with her and tried to help her orient herself. She would ask time and again how she got there, what she was doing there. Where was Dad? A couple of times she wondered if she had killed him! She wasn't particularly articulate, but I knew what she was asking. She thought that she had been such a burden to him that he had died from the strain of it. I said no. He had a bad heart. Actually, she had given him a reason to *live*. I would go through the whole thing. Dad got sick. You lived with John and me for the summer. Then you and Dad moved down here. Then Dad died of a heart attack. Now you are here near me. You are doing so well! I am so proud of you.

Mom would also hit the side of her head sometimes and sort of ask me what was wrong with her mind. She was becoming much less articulate, but she could still get an idea through. She could speak in short sentences, but anything resembling conversations were becoming rare. I would explain to her that she had Alzheimer's disease, and it made her forget things. She now accepted that truth.

She didn't quite understand the nature of the Cascade Inn. She would wonder why they wouldn't let her do any work. She was used to cooking, cleaning, and doing other work. Perhaps she would go back to teaching, she would say. Here again, in her mind she was a young woman. Once she passed a mirror and looked shocked at her reflection, exclaiming, "That isn't me!" Another time she said, "I don't know who that is!" This struck me as being *funny,* but it must have been horrifying for her to look in a mirror and not recognize the face looking back at her.

The routine at the Cascade Inn helped The Doctor Agnes, K.E. Meals and snacks were at the same time each day. Activities were from 10:00 A.M. until 3:00 P.M. She had a rest before dinner. There was a resident beautician who did Mom's hair each week. She had some lady friends she sat with.

One night around 10:00 P.M., the Inn called saying Mom was lost. I asked them to look again (my home was thirty minutes away) and call again in half-an-hour if she was still lost. She was found in a different room. She had a friend named Bea who also lost her husband of many years. Mother was in Bea's big double bed with her! This business of The Doctor going to bed with Bea ended up happening several times. I didn't care at all; they were both used to having a bed partner. It comforted them. The people who ran the Cascade Inn had their own agenda to follow, though.

One afternoon I came upon Mom when she was sitting alone. She was repeating over and over, *practicing,* "My name is Agnes Leonard. My name is Agnes Leonard. My name is Agnes Leonard." She wanted to remember her name, though all else was lost.

Mother lost some of her things at the Cascade Inn, the result of her taking things out of drawers constantly. She also seemed to acquire things. Once, I found a beautiful and expensive diamond watch among her things. Knowing it wasn't hers, I took it to the desk, and they located the owner. Another time The Doctor had a new, cute sweatshirt. Again I took it to the desk, but they never did find the owner, so Mom ended up with a new sweatshirt. Mom's wedding ring and other good jewelry should have been removed from her when we first moved her into the Inn. We could have told her we were going to have it cleaned or something—which indeed we could have done. There were many things left with Mom that we might have taken away for safekeeping. But we also wanted her to have her familiar things around her, so it was hard to find a balance. Still, it was a mistake not to take her rings, at the very least.

Some people have told me that nursing home staff and other institutional staff steal from residents. This probably does happen. My guess, having been around the mentally incompetent for a while, is that things get misplaced, lifted, borrowed, and so on by the residents themselves. Were I to do it over again, there would be many things I would have gradually removed from The Doctor's possession.

One of the first things I did after Dad died was to take Mom shopping for clothes. She needed just about everything! We bought her nighties, underwear, new shoes, a jacket and several warm-up type outfits—cute sweatshirts with matching sweat pants. Nearly everything was pink because that is what she liked and would wear.

Another priority was to take Mom to the dentist. She had always had soft teeth, which decayed easily, but her gums were beautiful. I had informed Dad from the beginning how important it was to see that Mom got regular medical and dental care. Alzheimer's victims lose the ability to express needs. Things like their vision, hearing, and teeth need to be checked regularly. An undetected decrease in vision and/or hearing can be dangerous. Not sure how long it had been since Mom had seen a dentist, and knowing her history, we took her in soon after Dad died. I have known our dentist since my college days when he was in dental school at the University of Washington. He later taught there as well. Trusting him completely, I made an appointment for The Doctor to have her teeth cleaned and examined. Heather actually was the one to take Mom in. Then I had a conference with the dentist, Dr. Richard (Dick) Moller. Dick told me that Mom's mouth was in poor condition, and he produced pictures as proof. He also had a machine where he could put a camera in Mom's mouth and have the picture projected on a screen. Mom's gums were abscessed and infected. Her teeth were rotting. Her bridgework was broken and loose. She needed one, maybe two root canals. It was quite a mess.

Dick said that basically we had two options. We could have her teeth pulled and get dentures for her, or we could spend several times as much money (he estimated over $6,000) and get everything fixed. I said I'd let him know.

In venting to Auntie Ethel, I told her I was so mad at Dad for letting Mom's teeth go, I would have shot him if he weren't already dead! Of course he had done the best he could, and he wasn't well. I just needed to rant and rave.

Both John and Tom were consulted for their advice. We reasoned that if we had Mom's teeth pulled and she got dentures, then she would surely lose them like she was losing everything else. If she had no teeth, she would have to eat soft foods only and would probably need nursing home care, just for the special diet. This would cost more than twice as much as the Cascade Inn. If we could keep her from a nursing home for just a few months, we could make up the money spent on fixing her teeth. So, while fixing her teeth looked expensive in the short run, nursing care resulting from dentures looked far more expensive in the long run.

I went back to Dick and explained to him that we had decided to fix Mom's teeth. However, since she didn't have a particularly long life-expectancy, he really didn't need to go with deluxe work. For example, where he might normally use a crown, if he thought a filling might last two or three years, he could go with the filling. Also he agreed to try to fix the bridges, rather than replacing them, but he couldn't promise it would work.

Thus began dental work that lasted for months. First, clean-up work had to be done with Mom's teeth and gums and time allowed for healing. Mom couldn't sit still in the chair for more than about 45 minutes, so she just had numerous appointments. For each of these, Ralph, Heather, Janelle, or I would sit and hold Mom's hand, stroking and comforting her.

Mom also had an appointment with Dr. Laderas, the internist who had treated Dad in the hospital and taken the time to get to know her patient. Mom had a flu shot and an exam, and we established Dr. Laderas as Mom's physician.

Wanting friends to be able to stay in touch with The Doctor Agnes, K.E., I sent out a form letter regarding her new life in Vancouver.

Dear Friends of Agnes Leonard,

This letter to you is from her daughter, Charlotte Akin. You all know that Dad passed away a few weeks ago. Many of you have asked about Mother, and I'm writing to fill you in.

Just over five years ago, Mother was diagnosed as having Alzheimer's Disease. She was diagnosed by the University of Washington in conjunction with Group Health. She has been part of the University's ongoing research for the past five years.

Some of you did not know that Mom has Alzheimer's. Dad was at first advised not to tell people because he and Mom could become social isolated. At first only immediate family knew. After a year or so, very close friends knew. Then the circle widened as it became more obvious and so forth. All along, one of the ironic reactions of people has been to be angry at the caregiver for suggesting anything was wrong with Mother. This is ironic because the fact that she can still present herself well in a social situation of three or more people is a direct result of the care she is getting!

Mother is at the beginning of the last stage of Alzheimer's. She does not ever really know where she is. She doesn't know the day, time of day, date, season, and so forth. She can bathe and dress herself with reminders and a little help. She hasn't been able to complete a task such as making a meal or sweeping a floor for over two years. She couldn't tell you the name of the president, my job, or any current event of any kind. But in a group of old friends (and the older the better!), she can carry on beautifully.

Dad's care of Mother was a thing of beauty. He fiercely defended her personhood. When the phone company was going to shut off the phone because Mom hadn't paid the bill, he continued to support her right to her checkbook and gradually began paying bills with her. When she could no longer drive because she got lost, he never told her to turn in her driver's license. In fact, it is current to this day. He did, however, sell her car! She was mad at him for a lifetime of buying and selling and trading. But he never let her think the car was sold because of a failure of *hers*. As Dad's health began to fail, he refused the orders of many doctors to put Mom in a nursing home or a foster home. He had seen her through the stages of depression, paranoia, anger, and madness that are part of Alzheimer's. As his health failed, Mom was entering a more docile stage. He moved with her to a retirement apartment near me in August.

Not all retirement apartments will take Alzheimer's patients, but we found one near the school where I teach. It has an Assisted Living wing, and the idea was that if anything happened to Dad, Mom could just move over there. Mom went to many activities in the Assisted Living wing right from the start. She liked their Bingo and exercise class. When Dad was hospitalized, I dropped Mom off in Assisted Living while I was at work and then brought her home with me overnight. The retirement apartment schedules some activities for the whole place, and some just for one side or the other. There's a beautiful shared courtyard, so many residents sit out and visit or eat outdoors. Each week there are scheduled trips out to shop, sight-see, etc. There are also many activities brought in—fashion shows, performances, and so forth. The last time Dad saw Mother, she was flushed and giddy as a school girl. She had had her hair done that day and had been square-dancing! She said she really cut loose! Dad literally shook his head and laughed at her. He passed away the next day; I moved Mom over to the Assisted Living wing the day after that.

So Mother is at the Cascade Inn, a *beautiful* retirement apartment complex of 160 residents, with a staff of 60. Because Dad managed to take care of her through the hostile and wandering stages, Mother is able to be in a beautiful place with no restraints. The staff—from the maintenance man to the cooks to the administrator—all watch her carefully. A kinder, more capable and caring staff you will never find. Mother has three good friends with whom she spends much of her day—Florence, Helen, and Bea. She even attempted to spend the night with Bea! She is awakened each morning, and her clothes are laid out. After breakfast there is exercise class. After lunch each day, there is a planned activity. After dinner there is Bingo, and on weekends there are complimentary movies. Mom gets her hair done once a week. We took her to see Dad after he passed away, and the memory was poignant enough for her to stop searching for him as she had done all summer while various members of the family cared for her because of Dad's health. She knows he is gone. She has some memory of him suffering and has said that because of this, she couldn't wish him back.

Mother loves to receive letters, phone calls, and visitors. She isn't able to reciprocate, but don't let that stop you!

> Thank you for your love and friendship,
> Charlotte

As the holidays approached, I thought of Mom's long-standing tradition of Thanksgiving with the Schmitts and the Binghams. Our family was going to Ralph's sister's home for Thanksgiving. It was out of the way, but we decided to drop Mom off at Homer and Betty's for one last time.

Mom spent Christmas with us, staying a night or two. It was astonishing how much her abilities had decreased since summer. She wasn't able to set a table, wrap a package, or write a sentence. She could sign her name, however, an ability that persisted long after other skills were gone. She was able to have only very short, barely coherent conversations. And only on really good days. She told me that Christmas that she couldn't forget Mary Lou and that was the one thing she wished she could! She also said, "I didn't do that right; I should have done that better." Giving her a pat, I said, "I know."

Late Dementia

The amount of care required for an Alzheimer's victim at this stage is enormous. Certainly, since the stage can last years, it is too much for an elderly spouse to handle alone. Decisions about care and about everything else are made by the caregiver alone. The Alzheimer's patient is unable to give meaningful input.

Verbal ability is lost at this stage. The person may become docile or difficult. Motor control declines. The person becomes incontinent of bladder and bowel. The ability to smile, walk, sit, chew, and swallow may all be lost. Certainly the ability to perform some or all of these tasks diminishes. The patient may need to be fed; he/she may refuse to eat. Eating difficulties raise ethical questions about forced feeding.

The Alzheimer's patient may become bedridden. As the brain becomes severely disrupted, the patient is more prone to seizures, infections, and so on. Inactivity increases the chances of pneumonia.

The Alzheimer's victim experiences eventual stupor and coma leading to death (Gruetzner, 1988).

Chapter 9

Assisted Living
Early 1992

John and Denise came down to see Mom, bringing Natalie and Andrew. The Cascade Inn is a deluxe retirement apartment complex. It has lovely common areas both indoors and outdoors. Inside, the walls are hung with beautiful, classical prints as well as homey touches, such as wreaths. It is immaculately clean and always decorated seasonally. The common rooms have fireplaces, sofas, chairs, and books. One large wing housing around 200 residents is for independent retirees. A smaller wing, housing perhaps thirty, is for assisted living. It was to this wing that John's family went in search of The Doctor. Apparently, John walked right past Mom, and she did not know him. Not expecting this, John was jolted. The whole family was upset by the visit. They weren't used to seeing Mom out of her own home. They were struck by the fact that, however nice it was, Granny was in an institution. It might have helped if I had been there.

I was learning to give The Doctor Agnes, K.E., visual clues to help her *and me* when I came. I would always do something to get her attention and then I would give her a big, "so *nice* to see you!" smile. She would smile back, and we would both feel good. The Doctor used to say with a baby "you just smile a smile into him." She meant that a baby learned to smile by being smiled at. Indeed, most people smile when they are smiled at. A victim of Alzheimer's, being somewhat "empty" like a new baby, will give back what is given. They must be smiled at to smile back.

John isn't the big smile type. He isn't an actor. Putting on a smile when he was worried or sad was an unnatural act. He hadn't the experience of knowing how to get the best out of Mom. If he looked concerned, it made

The Doctor feel anxious, worried. This is what he got back. So visiting her was much harder for him from many angles. He did appreciate my skill in dealing with Mom.

I got a letter from Aunt Babe telling me how wonderful I am. John and Tom both appreciated my care of The Doctor and seemed to let others know it. It was oh-so-nice to have the support.

From a letter written back to Aunt Babe dated January 1992:

No, I'm not sprouting wings and a halo yet! Tom and family are due down next weekend. We'll have Mom out here Friday and Saturday. I think it'll be easier for them to see her here. John felt so sad when he saw Mom last time. Her mind is slipping steadily away. She hasn't had so much as a cold this winter though....

Dad apparently didn't get her into the dentist the past several years, and she needs between $5-8,000 worth of dental work—or dentures, which she'd lose...without teeth she'd be in a nursing home in no time, and I'm committed to avoiding that if at all possible. But I'm not a Genie—she could land there anyway if other things come along. In spite of this, Mom seems fine—still is capable of enjoying whatever moment she is living in. I'll go in to see her after school tomorrow. I always take her bananas and hard candy and her laundry. I'll stay for dinner with her. Janelle has a piano lesson, so we'll all get home around 7:00. Homer and Betty are heading south on Thurs. and stopping at Mom's.

My second graders are my therapy. It's hard to think of oneself with twenty-three seven-year-olds demanding attention!

I talked to Auntie Ethel last weekend. She is heading to Phoenix where she'll meet up with Homer and Betty, Homer's brother, and some others. Then she wants to go to Vegas to put some closure on the passing of Dad and Uncle Harold. [Dad had "won" the bet with Uncle Harold, beating him to the Pearly Gates by about two months.] *I guess there's a group in Vegas they (Mom and Dad and Harold and Ethel) always saw. Anyhow, I think she'll be OK—she's a dear person.*

I don't know the best time to tell you to call Mom. Probably

Saturday mornings. She is involved in activities on week-days—exercise class each morning, and after lunch Bingo or van rides or crafts, ice cream and popcorn socials, etc. The dining room is one end of a "great room" with a big TV, tables to sit around, and sofas and easy chairs by the fireplace. She goes to meals and activities out there and stays to visit. Except for Sunday church, her weekends are free; she often naps in the afternoon. So Saturday mornings you might catch her! She is not able to structure her day, to complete any meaningful task anymore. She can't write a letter or anything. This routine fills her days, and she just lives in the moment. As long as the moment is nice—people are nice to her, her surroundings are pretty, and so forth—she is fine. Once in a while she will remember that she has lost Dad, and then she is sad. But she's very easily distracted from that. The staff gets her up in the morning and calls her to meals and activities. If she gets bored, she tells me that she is going back to work. She seems aware that she no longer works. While she was at home she was quite sure she was keeping house, fixing meals etc. She's not used to feeling unproductive. I always tell her I'll put her to work at my house. We do let her dig in the garden, help fix a salad—anything so she feels she's chipping in.

Mom's life at the Cascade Inn did have some ups and downs. She was forever taking her pictures off her walls and taking them apart. This she added to the uproar of her drawers and closets. Once, she called Homer and Betty long distance from another resident's room and told them to come and get her! Most of the time, this kind of action was beyond her capabilities. Now and then she could remember things like a phone number, or realize that she was not at her own home. The Inn did not at that time have any security on the outside doors. Although she would have to go some distance from either her room or the dining/activity area to get outside the compound, it could be done. She could go outdoors into a garden with lawns and eating area right off her dining room. But it didn't go anywhere. She was safe there. We looked into security systems, but they had to be wired into the institution. She seemed to be past her real wandering days, so we had to weigh that risk with a loss of freedom for her.

Also, Mom felt like she was in a hotel at the Inn. She didn't feel like she was at home. This was not expressed directly as she was losing the ability to do that. She would say, "I have no work to do." She would usually be wearing her coat, as though she were going somewhere, or wanted to. She wondered why she had no money. I would always put a little of my spare change in her purse, and of course she lost it. It made her feel better. Often she would try to sleep with Bea.

Mother was raised in a good Norwegian family. She was taught not to complain. She would say to me, "Well, you know I never complain." Then I was left to wonder what she might want to complain about! She also told me once quite plainly while she was at the Inn, "I don't know what I'd do now without you."

During this period, Mom was "in" her teens. She would ask when she was going to get to see her parents. (When she went to high school she had to board with a family near the high school, so she missed her family.)

It was hard for Mom to grieve the loss of Dad since she kept forgetting that he had died. Occasionally she would say, "Did he die? or "He died, didn't he?" It was a faint knowing. Just once I found her in her room crying for him.

When I took Mom out, men would look her over. She looked pretty cute for a 75-year-old woman. Once she was mad and talked about that "vile old man!" thinking of herself as much younger.

We brought Mom home for all holidays with us. At Easter she told me in a girlish way, "I don't have to help because my dress is too pretty." She was making a joke, like a child trying to get out of chores. She saw hummingbirds come to our feeder and was fascinated. "Are they real?" she asked. Reality was becoming lost to her. She told me the post tops on our deck, which she could see from the kitchen window, were "the heads of little children looking in at us." She thought my home was a resort or a vacation place, undoubtedly because of its location in a forest. In addition to these delusions, she was also beginning to mumble.

As The Doctor's mental condition deteriorated, her placement at the Cascade Inn became less and less appropriate. However, *that was not what it felt like at the time to me.* To me it felt as if people weren't doing their jobs. I kept having to go to the Inn to take care of things. Little things, big things, all kinds of things. The dentist Mom was seeing regularly was telling me that her teeth weren't getting brushed. That kind of help was available at the Cascade Inn in the Assisted Living Wing. Indeed, we were paying for it. The aides were being instructed to brush Mom's teeth. But Mom would say, "Oh, I can do that," or "I've already brushed my teeth," and it wouldn't get done. She could still fool people into thinking she could do more than she really could. Also, since there were shifts of people—most of them minimum wage, and some of them part time—it might be several different people each week to brush her teeth, for example. They didn't catch on. Mom could go a whole week with only one pair of dirty under-pants in the laundry. She was wearing things over and over again. She was even sleeping in her clothes. Again, she was fooling the people who were supposed to dress her. To the night person she might say, "I can get ready for bed myself." Then the night person would lay out her clothes for bed and her clothes for the next day. In the morning when the next shift was on, the aide would come in and say, "Oh, I see you are already dressed," while actually she was still wearing yesterday's clothes. Because the toothbrush and toothpaste were left out, the aide might ask, "Have you already brushed your teeth, too?" And Mom would say, "Yes!" Mom *looked* like she was a capable person. At the Inn very few of their people needed this kind of care. The aides were not particularly trained in it. Although it didn't seem so at the time, the problem was not the Inn. It was Mother's placement there as her Alzheimer's worsened.

Chapter 10

Transitions
Spring and Summer 1992

One evening I stopped by late after school to see The Doctor. I had worked late, past 7:00 P.M. Mom was already in bed. It was a Friday night. Ralph had left on a trip to Siberia the day before. He was going on a business visa with a group from his Rotary Club. Janelle was gone for the night. I just wanted to pick up Mom's laundry, check in on her, and go home. On my way out, I stopped to talk with one of the staff. She asked if I knew that Mom had gotten out this week. No, I didn't know. She mentioned that there was some kind of record or notation of times this had happened. She said that Mom had gotten into a neighborhood across a busy street. A stranger had looked at her ID bracelet and brought her back. I thanked the nurse and left.

The next morning I was able to contact the head nurse in Assisted Living to get more details. It seemed that this had happened twice before. They were keeping a record so they could let me know if it was happening at the same time each day or just on weekends when there was no activity routine, and so on.

All of this jolted me. I had weighed the possibility of Mom getting lost because she was not in a "secure" (lock-up) facility against the loss of freedom she'd have in a nursing home. I decided it was a risk worth taking. I had a good friend in a nursing home and another who administered one, so I was familiar with their services. I had even weighed The Doctor being in the Inn against the more remote possibility of her getting hit by a car if she ever got out and decided that also was still a risk worth taking, but just barely. Like Dad, I placed a high value on freedom and quality of life, sometimes higher even than safety. What I hadn't thought of was the risk of her being taken by someone and abused. We couldn't count on every stranger who found her being good-hearted. The risk of abduction and abuse was not a risk worth taking. Mother was docile enough at this point to go along with anyone who took her hand. Now she had figured out how to get out and was doing it repetitively! I went to the Inn, packed a bag for her, and took her home with me.

Of course I struggled again with whether to bring The Doctor home to live with my family. Auntie Ethel was steadfast in reminding me that this was *not* what Mom would have wanted. Aunt Babe said the same. What a gift it was to me that Mom spoke of this years before and was resolute that she did not want to live with her children, no matter what. What she had said was that she did not want to burden her family. I'm not sure we get to choose that. Certainly her care was a burden. But Auntie Ethel had taken her own mother in and she knew what a change in lifestyle to everyone that was. Janelle and Ralph, Homer and Betty—all were in agreement that it would not be best to bring The Doctor home.

That morning I needed to get new tires on my car. While Mom and I were waiting, I made some calls. I called a nursing home that had a good reputation, but the administrator wasn't available at the moment. Could I call back in the afternoon? Then I picked up a newspaper, remembering Dad's visit to the foster care home with his friend from the Alzheimer's Support Group. I looked in the want ads for foster care. I finally found some listings for "Adult Care" and called one. The line was busy. I called another, Annabelle's Foster Care. The lady, a registered nurse, said that Annabelle was not there but that I could stop by for a look, and she would give me some references. She told me that they had experience with Alzheimer's. Since it was on my way home and my car was just about done, I said we'd be right over.

The home was in a nice, middle-class neighborhood. It was a fairly typical three-bedroom, two-bathroom rancher with a double garage. It had a fenced yard with roses along the border. Inside, the home was soft and clean. Very clean. It smelled like homemade cooking. The walls were a soft peach. Wallpaper in the bedrooms were also in the soft pastels that The Doctor loved. The nurse who was there had her two kids with her, and they had a puppy. It was a home full of life and fun. An older lady, named Belle, sat having coffee at the dining room table with her visiting daughter amidst this. They both told me what a wonderful home it was. Belle had a cancer surgery that left her with a colostomy. She was sharp as a tack and sweet. She had lived there over two years. Another lady there was bedridden, had Parkinson's, and her mind was also gone. Mom and I went out on the deck through sliding glass doors just off the dining room. We walked in the fenced back yard. Then I got the references and took Mom home with me.

Laying The Doctor down for a nap, I called the references. Some had people there for a year or more. Not a single negative comment was heard. Annabelle Beatty Rhodes, the owner, was wonderful and loving. The food was good. Everyone was clean and happy. And on. And on.

Saturday evening I called Annabelle and told her that I wanted to move The Doctor in. With Janelle sitting with Mom, I went back over to Annabelle's, filled out some paperwork for her, and told her I would bring Mom the next day, moving most of Mom's things on Monday.

(It should be noted that I paid both Heather and Janelle minimum wage for errands and "baby-sitting" that they did for Mom out of The Doctor's checking account. While they hadn't asked for it, I felt it was only fair. When I consulted Tom and John, they felt the same. We all knew what a lot of work this was.)

So Sunday, The Doctor moved into Annabelle's. It was the third time I had moved her in under eight months. Of course I felt guilty. Mom hardly knew her own name, and I kept moving her around!

On Monday most of the rest of Mom's things were moved out of the Inn. Connie, the administrator, let me store some things there for a short time—such as furniture that Ralph could help me deal with when he got home from Russia.

On Tuesday I got sick. I was treated for strep, but I didn't get well. After two weeks and a couple of different antibiotics, the clinic did a mononucleosis test on me, even though 44-year-olds do not normally get mono. I had it. Had I been under any unusual stress?

Far too sick to see Mom, I phoned, sent Janelle, or sent Ralph. I got well enough after a few more weeks to go back to work where I got sick again. In between was Mother's Day. Ralph was again out of town. Janelle and I took The Doctor to the Mongolian Grill for dinner, a place we all liked. It was the first time I had to feed Mom. Otherwise, she just sat there and wouldn't eat. She lacked motivation, lacked initiative.

Getting through the remainder of the school year in fits and starts, I felt it had also been a rough year for my class. At the beginning of the year their teacher had been gone for a death in the family, and at the end, she was gone because of mono.

John came that spring to check in on Mom. It was so hard for him to see her. The worse her mind got, the harder it was for him. We took her on a little walk. He could see that she had good care. But he was so saddened by the visit.

Both Tom's and John's families offered to take Mom and place her in Alaska and Idaho respectively, to relieve me. It was so good to have the offers and the support. They understood clearly the strain I'd been under; their offers were an acknowledgment of that. I gave it serious consideration.

Over the summer I would drop in at various times of the day to see The Doctor in her new home, often unannounced. While I respected the fact that this was a home, not an institution, I had responsibility for The Doctor's care. So at first I visited frequently. It was interesting sometimes to see what The Doctor Agnes, K.E. brought with her—what parts of her personality persisted. One day there was a cup in the kitchen windowsill with a rose in it, something she'd done all the time at her home in Seattle. Another time she was on the sofa with about three rollers in her hair, kind of here and there— another familiar scene.

Sometimes The Doctor came home with me for a day. She enjoyed picking berries, walking, and listening to Heather play old hymns on the piano for her. She could even remember the words to some of them and would hum the tune for many.

When Mom began to lose weight, I brought her home with me for a day and fixed all of her favorite foods. She barely touched them. Often she would say that her stomach was upset, but she wasn't sick, depressed, or anxious. Once, thinking of herself as much younger, she told Annabelle that she thought she was pregnant! When I took Mom, Janelle, and friends to the ocean for a day, Mom ate ice cream and little else. She even refused clam chowder, her favorite. The Doctor Agnes, K.E., lost 27 pounds in 1992. Never able to pinpoint the cause, we all wondered how long she would last at that rate. Annabelle—whom I was now calling "Ann"—began giving Mom Ensure, a nutritional supplement in the form of puddings and shakes.

Once on a drive, The Doctor gave me a clear-eyed look. She was still occasionally able to get ideas through purposefully and sometimes she would give me this look, and I would know to pay attention; she had something to say. This time she said, "The mother there is good." I said, "Yes. You mean Ann. She is very good to you, and she is good at what she does." Mom nodded. As I learned to trust Ann and her care of Mom, I could let go of some of it. And I needed to for my own health and the health of my family. Mom was getting excellent one-on-one care. I knew by the end of the summer that we didn't need to move her to Idaho or Alaska.

I wrote again to Mother's friends and relatives:

Dear Friends and Relatives of Agnes Leonard,

I moved Mom the first of April to a foster home. It was becoming increasingly obvious that she needed more personal attention than she was getting at the Assisted Living wing of the retirement apartments. We had believed that Mom moved out of the wandering stage of her disease ages ago. But when the nice weather came, she really just had to go out in it. She got lost big-time twice and was developing a pattern of leaving, so I brought her home with me for a weekend, and we found a foster home for her. It has a fenced, locked back yard, so that she can go outdoors any time. She can water or hose off the deck. The first thing she did after we moved her was to get a little sunburn!

There are two other ladies at the foster home. And there is a couple who lives there. The woman, Ann, has done this kind of work for several years, and she has had Alzheimer's people before. Ann also employs an RN full-time who is on call as well on week-ends and evenings.

Mother is very child-like now. She likes to help Ann. She drinks her milkshake first if we take her out for dinner. She often thinks she is in South Dakota.

One of the nicest things about Mom's new place is that if friends or family call her, she is actually around to take a call! Mid-morning and dinner time are good times to call.

If you are stopping by to see Mom, give Ann a call, and she can tell you easy directions. Mom may not remember if you call or come and see her, but she does have a *sense* of anything repetitive. She has a niece and nephew that send a card once a week. And Mom will say, "Now haven't they been nice to me?' Or I might say, "Have you had any calls?" And she'll say, "Yes, I think I have." I've just put together a photo album for her with pictures that go as far back as I could find. Mom loves to look at the old photos. She even loves old news! When I told her that her sister-in-law, Lilian, had married Cecil Milner, she hooted in delight, "No kidding?!" I'm sure they've been married over 30 years. So even though Mom may not be able to reciprocate or make very much sense, calls, letters, pictures, visits, and so on do connect her to her world, and she does *feel* that.

Mom still looks great. To look at her, one still cannot tell that there is anything wrong. Her walk is very slow now and sometimes a little unsteady. But she still has her rosy complexion and a smile. She remains determined to not be a complainer, to make the best of every situation. It amazes me the fine threads of character that remain . . . that usually are not even visible, and then the light hits them a certain way, and sure enough, one can see them; they are still there.

> Keep in touch,
> Charlotte

Ann had all kinds of nifty tricks to help The Doctor. She would tuck Mom into bed at night and give her a kiss. This somehow seemed to help Mom stay in bed. I mentioned it to a friend who was caring for her own mother who also suffered from a dementing illness. It worked for her, too. Mom was so *busy* and *messy* that living with her was difficult. She was much worse than a house full of preschoolers because she couldn't remember anything. It wasn't possible to make things off limits to her. Closets, cupboards, drawers, purses—all were within her reach and interest. She couldn't be punished for misbehaving because it would do no good, and she wouldn't know what she had done. It's not legal to confine or lock a patient in a room in a foster care home because of fire danger. (My friend's mother, cared for at home, had a Dutch door installed in her bedroom doorway. She could be confined to the room, but still be part of the family with the top part open.) But Ann did have some tricks. She used some of the safety devices on cupboards and doors that work for preschoolers. She also put very little in drawers in The Doctor's room and bathroom. Some might even be empty or just contain things Mom liked to play with like cards, letters from friends, picture albums. We had to take pictures off the walls for a while because she kept taking them down and taking them apart. Flowered wallpaper still made the room look decorated. Ann's back yard was fenced and locked, so The Doctor had freedom back there. The deck also had a lock on it. Sometimes Ann cared for people for whom stairs were difficult, so the lock on the deck was for them. Ann also knew that Mom could brush her own teeth better than anyone else. Ann would get their toothbrushes out and ready, and they would brush *together*. Ann might watch and check to see that they were getting done; she might also brush Mom's teeth. Getting Mom to do it herself was a very effective way of getting the job done—and it worked for *years*! (We—Ralph, Heather, Janelle, or I—took The Doctor in for professional dental cleaning quarterly. The reports were that her gums were much improved.)

The relationship that developed between The Doctor and Ann was a thing of beauty. Ann was cute and shapely, and she loved a good time. They actually had these things in common. Ann loved it when Mom made a little joke. Mom loved it when Ann dressed up, when she laughed, fixed her hair, danced a little with her. It had never occurred to me that The Doctor was able to make new friends at this stage of her life and disease, but I watched it happen with Ann. Mom trusted Ann almost from the first day. And Ann had a respect for Mom that made me stop and think. Ann respected the fact that Mom made an effort to be loving. She could see that The Doctor worked at being good. Mom let Ann know in many ways how much she appreciated Ann. She would tell her so each night at bedtime. That a person entering the late stages of Alzheimer's could win the respect of other people was profoundly enlightening to me. I knew that *I* felt that way about The Doctor, but I had watched her battle this disease from the beginning. That The Doctor could make a *new* friend, could win *new* respect, love a *new* person was something I hadn't thought of as being possible. Yet in a very little while, Ann and The Doctor were as close as the closest friends. They worked and played together and enjoyed each other.

I made it a point from before I introduced Dad and The Doctor to Connie at the Inn to never tell others any negative details about my parents. First, every family has its horror stories. Second—and more important—I wanted the best care for Mom and Dad. I did not want to color a caregiver's perception of either of my parents by accenting the negative. Their care was at least partly my responsibility. To get the best, I wanted to help them put their best foot forward, so to speak. This practice was so worthwhile, even for me. The love and fun between Ann and The Doctor made my visits a joy.

Mother shared a room that first summer with Ann's mother-in-law, the bedridden woman we had met on our first visit. The elder Mrs. Rhodes had been placed with Ann. This was how her son, Ken, came to know Ann. Ken and Ann were married just a few months before I placed The Doctor with Ann.

In another break with reality, Mother referred to the elder Mrs. Rhodes as "that cute little girl." Mom would kind of fuss over her. The Doctor would also read to her. If The Doctor lost her place, she would just start again at the top of the page. Surely "that cute little girl" heard some pages of the *Reader's Digest* hundreds of times!

Mom was also allowed to "help" Ann. She could go out again to "her own" rose garden. She could dig in dirt or water flowers. Ann would put Mother on the sofa with a pile of clean laundry to "fold." She might be given a wet rag when Ann washed the kitchen floor. The Doctor Agnes, K.E., would clean one small area over and over while Ann cleaned the whole kitchen. Mom no longer wanted to put her coat on. She was past most of her packing stage. She was home.

A new resident, a man named Victor, had had a stroke. Victor liked to dance, too, so he and The Doctor would occasionally entertain others by dancing together. Ken's father had been a music professor; there was often music playing. One day Mom went into Victor's room only to come flying out a few minutes later saying, "That bastard!" We never did find out what he did to offend her. But it didn't diminish their dancing. It's difficult to hold a grudge when one can't remember what happened from one minute to the next.

Taking Mom to the doctor was a "happening." In the waiting room she liked the pictures of babies in *Parents* magazine. If there were real babies in the waiting room, that was even better. Mom was delighted. Dr. Laderas wanted her to have a mammogram since she was on estrogen. *Doing* this was another matter. Most women can barely put up with it when they understand fully why it needs to be done, and how it will be done. Still, it's nobody's idea of a good time. For someone without the capacity to understand, it's challenging in previously unimagined ways. The Doctor Agnes, K.E., was in no way happy with having a stranger manipulate her breasts. Then there was the procedure known as the "urine specimen." Mom was not amused by me trying to take down her pants. She could not understand why I needed to have my hand in her crotch with a cup when she was on the toilet! Going to the bathroom on command was also out of her league. So we would go for a ride, stopping off for a large root beer float, and then traipse back to the doctor's office for another try.

While The Doctor didn't like her pants down in the rest room, taking them down in *other* places seemed like a good idea to her. When I took her to the beach, she kept trying to pull her pants down to scratch an itch on her bottom. It was all I could do to keep them on her. Eating in restaurants was getting awkward. She would sometimes play with her food. She might break up a roll and drop the pieces in her coffee. She might pick up her water glass and empty it on the table. It was like having an unruly two-year-old on my hands, the difference being that a two-year-old could reason and follow directions. Trips to the rest room were frustrating. If I went in a stall, who was watching The Doctor? She would leave the area! If she was in a stall, I would either have to hold the door or take my chances with her locking it from the inside. It actually took *three* people to use a public rest room—if Mom was one of them. Taking her out in public was becoming more difficult because her behavior was not always appropriate. *Most* of the time it was still all right.

For Mom's 76th birthday the bridge club, as well as Homer and Betty and a few long-time friends, came to my house. Many expressed feelings of guilt for not seeing Mom since Dad had died, but she wasn't easy to visit one-on-one for most people. It was easier to see her with a group of others, especially in a party setting. This was better for everyone anyway. Mom had a great time, even remembering a few names. Of course their faces were still familiar to her.

Still quite weak in the summer from my bout with mono, I wasn't sure if I could teach. Our daughter Heather was in college, so it would have been a financial strain without me teaching. I considered bringing Mom to our home, not for the first or last time. I would charge the estate for her care and that would be my income. Again both my family and my aunts advised against it. So did all my friends. Janelle was the deciding factor. She was dead set against it, saying she'd go live with a friend. Ralph asked what he could do to help me. I said, "Do the shopping!" So Ralph did the shopping from then on.

In the crazy busyness of working and taking care of Mom and Dad, a long habit of daily walking had gotten lost. I committed to regular walking again both for strength as well as a stress-reliever. I went back to work and gradually got stronger.

Other changes in my life took shape that summer, some the result of mono, some the result of The Doctor being with Ann, some because it was time. I went back to Seattle to see the home where I had spent part of my childhood. We were renting the house out to a family with four children. I asked if they minded if I just walked through. They gave their permission. The house was again clean and full of fun. The children were well behaved; there was laughter. Windows were open letting in the cool salt breeze from the beach. The raspberries were ripe, the fuchsias in bloom. It was a better goodbye than the party after Dad's funeral or the day we moved them out. I was glad I had gone.

Once school started up, I only visited Mom regularly once a week. Gone were the days of tending her morning and night. I often saw her more than once in a given week. But I didn't *need* to. And since I'd had to spend so much time resting, I began to write about The Doctor, keeping a journal on her and making a commitment to write on a 5x7 card about her each time I visited. In the lingo of a scientist, these were actually field notes. It dawned on me that there was a lot of data on The Doctor already. For years I had kept notes in the margins of copies from books I'd made describing the course of the disease. There were copies of some of the monthly reports we sent to the University of Washington. I had copies of letters to friends and relatives. My own personal journal had some documentation. I was able to step back mentally and see my mother as a valuable case study. This was an *interesting* disease which had stricken a woman with the dogged and selfless courage to allow herself to be repeatedly exposed to humiliating testing in the hope of helping others she would never know. Helpless now, might it be worthwhile to carry on for her? I began to think about telling her story.

Chapter 11

Fall and Winter 1992

Ann's husband, Ken, was a quiet man. With a doctorate from Columbia University, he had spent some time as a history teacher. But he had left academia to become an electrician. In addition, he helped with a variety of chores for Ann's business.

Mom really liked Ken. (In truth, she really liked men, telling Ann that she thought she'd look for another man.) She flirted often with Ken, and I would tease Ann, warning her that she'd better keep an eye on them. Once Mom told Ann, "I wish there was one more of him." Another time when Ken came home from work, The Doctor jumped up, went over to him, put her arms around his neck, kissed him on the mouth and said, "Happy New Year!" Ken is a reserved and consummately polite gentleman; he was left speechless by this. Ann thought it was hysterical, particularly since it happened in October.

Beautiful fall days often beckoned to The Doctor and me for a drive to a nearby farm, where we'd end up buying anything from fresh honey to ornamental pumpkins for Mom's room. Two such places were not far from the foster care home, Joe's Place and Kunze Farms. Both had produce stands as well as working farms. Often we'd buy a treat, apple cider, or fresh produce to take back and share. Mom always liked the out-of-doors, and this never really changed.

We did have to be careful with her, though, because she was becoming more easily chilled. I bought her some long underwear, and that helped. She wore it under her sweaters or sweatshirts and under her slacks or sweat pants. Hats and mittens also became part of her wardrobe, and she wore these on our outings together any time the temperature was under about 60 degrees.

Fall meant a trip to Dr. Laderas for a flu shot, not only for Mom, but also as a courtesy for those with whom she lived. John, Tom, and I talked about the ethics of Mom's care often. Did avoidance of the flu prolong her life? Homer and Betty stopped down periodically, and I also visited with them by phone. They had taken care of the wife of one of Homer's colleagues when she was in a nursing home for years after Homer's colleague had passed away. They were familiar with the issues facing us. While we wouldn't do anything to unnaturally prolong Mom's life—no heroics—we decided that reasonable preventive medicine was acceptable. We did have a DNR (do not resuscitate) order put on Mom in case of a catastrophic event such as a heart attack or stroke. Ann and Dr. Laderas were both given copies of the order. Here again, it was consistent with how *I* would want to be treated, and it was what Mother had said she wanted back in the days when her brain was in order.

After an outing or a visit to the doctor, Mom would want to follow me home. Alzheimer's patients tend to bond to one or two people. They will follow that person around, look to that person for direction, and so on. This is another reason why foster care is a good alternative for them. As lovely as the Cascade Inn was, there were too many shifts of people for The Doctor to firmly bond to one. The closest she came there was with the Assisted Living Activity Director. Sometimes when I left The Doctor to go home, she would want to come with me. Once she was in foster care, she bonded beautifully to Ann, too. I could tell her, "Oh, I think Ann needs you to help her fix dinner now." Then I'd turn her around or turn her attention to Ann who played along, and Mom would go with her.

Sometimes Mom really did help Ann. My October 30th journal entry:

Ann said Mom made a salad last week—she still wants to work. Peeled and chopped up bananas and apples and then chopped up some banana nut bread. Ann thought she'd have to feed it to the birds, but it tasted pretty good so they added whipped cream and raisins and had it for dinner! Mom told Ann, "I've still got it!"

Ann is going to let the ladies stay up late tomorrow to see the trick or treaters. Mom looked great—cozy and happy.

By the time I had taken care of Mom for a year, I realized that we hadn't heard a peep from the University of Washington. Knowing that she had been tested annually, I finally got back in contact with Meredith Pfanschmidt, the study coordinator. She said that Dad had terminated The Doctor's participation when they made the move to Vancouver because he didn't want to burden me. One of the conditions of the study was an agreement for the subject to be autopsied shortly after death. Dad didn't want me to have that hassle. But I also knew two things. First, longitudinal (long-term) research is compromised most often by the loss of subjects over time. This is a valuable, difficult, and expensive form of research. The results, however, can lose validity if too many people drop out of the study over time. Second, The Doctor so wanted to make a contribution. I asked Meredith if Mom could be reinstated. She agreed, saying that not too much time had elapsed.

On October 30th Sam Lashley, a psychometrist, came from the University of Washington to test The Doctor. I also had the chance to ask him some questions on the phone. Because of specifications having to do with grant money and other technicalities, people at the University of Washington could not share actual data with me. They could answer general questions about Mom and about Alzheimer's, though. We had copies of some of the reports on The Doctor that we'd sent in regularly for years.

Asking Sam about personality changes in this stage of the disease, he said that some people are the same as always—only more so! Others are completely different from what they were. This phenomenon seems to be random, or else it is not known why some change and some are similar to their former selves. Their care is not known to be a factor. About Mom, Sam said that her regression had gone at an even pace. She had declined at a steady rate. This was a comfort to me because we all worried that The Doctor had declined so much since Dad died. I worried that moving her had caused decline. Sam had test results over several years that showed the rate of her change to be about the same. With Dad gone and in new surroundings, she couldn't as easily hide the disease. Also she was at a point in the course of Alzheimer's that is difficult to disguise because so *much* ability had been lost. Sam also said Mom was considerably happier than when he had last seen her. That had been in her Seattle home when she was crying over Dad's "unfaithfulness" and was generally depressed. All of this made me feel better about taking care of Mom.

The Doctor's appetite picked up again finally in the fall. Periods of no appetite alternated with periods of good appetite for the rest of her days. When she was eating well, Ann just fed her large portions and often. When her appetite was gone, she went back on Ensure. Frequently on a drive I would take Mom to the drive-through at McDonald's or Dairy Queen for an ice cream treat. She could still make a choice, once asking for "a-er-a split." I got her a banana split, and she ate the whole thing! Butterscotch sundaes were also a favorite. When she got so that she couldn't tell me anymore, I just knew I had a sure bet with either a "split" or a sundae.

Incontinence began with just a few widely separated events. Usually Ann could tell when Mom needed to use the bathroom, just by watching her. Mom would look uncomfortable or hold herself, much like a very young child. Ann also had Mother on a very regular bathroom schedule. At this point, too, The Doctor Agnes, K.E., could usually tell and get herself to the bathroom, if she could find it. The Doctor was embarrassed by her accidents. But Ann always treated her with respect and love, acting as if this was no big deal. Sometimes Ann would find that Mom had rinsed out her underpants. Mother was meticulously clean about herself, and this never changed. To the end of her days Ann would say, "She's always a lady." I suggested diapers for The Doctor long before Ann wanted to use them. Ann had a sense about when a person would accept this, and so she waited, covering her furniture with attractive throws that hid a waterproof pad. Her home always smelled as clean as mine did!

Mom also began speaking in Norwegian. As a child she didn't speak English at all until she was five years old and went to school. In her early sixties, she and her South Dakota chum, Mabel Patterson, left their husbands and took off for Norway together. By that time she was sure she had forgotten how to speak Norwegian entirely, but when she got to Norway she found it came flooding back. She could speak it like a five-year-old, talking about things like food and family. She didn't have enough to talk politics or any other adult topic. Now, as part of her regression into the past, she began speaking Norwegian occasionally. Once at our house when we sat down for dinner she said grace in Norwegian! Ann told me she sounded as if she was saying sentences in Norwegian from time to time.

Speaking in Norwegian was part of Mom's journey back in time. Her demeanor at this time was that of a teenager. She flirted with men, especially Ken and Ralph. Her own family of Babe, Dagny, and her brothers, was on her mind far more than the family she and Dad built. If asked her age, she might say "fifteen." The youngest age she could ever tell us was twelve. After that, she lost the ability to answer a direct question except for "yes" or "no."

It's also possible that this regression into Norwegian was precipitated by the arrival of a new helper for Ann. Ana, a Romanian immigrant who lived across the street, was trained by Ann to fill in for her. Ana came in the mornings often bringing her two little girls with her. Mother was thrilled. She had always loved children, and now she had two to play with. She undoubtedly heard Ana speaking Romanian to her girls. Perhaps this sparked Mother's recall of Norwegian. The Doctor taught the girls a little Norwegian dance. They actually played together.

Mother knew she was losing her mind, I'm convinced, all along. Earlier in the disease when she sent away for Alzheimer's information, then the terrible depressions, practicing "My name is Agnes Leonard" at the Inn, hitting the side of her head and saying something was wrong—these were all indications that she *knew* and that she *worked* at retaining her mind. One day at Ann's she said very mechanically, "My name is Agnes Leonard, but I don't know anything else." It sounded rehearsed.

It seemed that little problems were a way of life with The Doctor. We'd get one solved when another would pop up. The Doctor took to tying knots in her shoe laces. Not a knot or two, but as many knots as could be tied! Ann said she was spending hours untying knots. So we looked for shoes with Velcro, but as luck would have it, just when Mom needed it, it was no longer in style. We even checked Goodwill and other second hand stores. Finally, Ralph and I found some on a Christmas shopping trip.

Then, suddenly, Mom started getting up and dressed after she had been put to bed—even with her hug and kiss. She was also agitated in the evenings, wanting to leave. I suggested that Ann give The Doctor her desipramine earlier in the day, perhaps at dinner rather than bedtime. This was a medication with a sedative effect that she had been on for emotional problems since her wild days with Dad. The change worked well. Ann and I share the same philosophy about medications. We like to use the fewest possible and the least amount. The Doctor had been taken off estrogen, so desipramine was the only medication she was on. After working with Ann for a while, I began to tell her that she could use the medicine however it worked best. I had talked it over with Dr. Laderas, who was prescribing the desipramine in 25 mg tablets. Mom could have up to 75 mg per day. Throughout Mom's long illness, we varied the medication as her needs and moods changed. Sometimes she needed none, sometimes we split the dosage, morning and evening. If Mom had to go to the dentist, doctor, or beauty shop, we might give her a pill just before she left to calm her. More often than not The Doctor needed only 25 mg per day. Ann was so skilled with Mom, and she was with her so much, that it only made sense to give her some freedom with Mom's care.

While The Doctor's ability to converse was nearly gone, she could still *think, react, and feel.* She could still *communicate.* After one day out together, for example, she was mumbling along on the way home, and I heard her say, "apple." A minute or two later out popped "fruit." When we got home to Ann I told her, "I think Mom is hungry for some fruit. So Ann set a bowl of sliced peaches in front of her which she ate—and then polished that off with a piece of carrot cake! From my journal dated November 19, 1992:

> When I got there today I asked her if she wanted to go for a ride. She no longer verbalizes well, but she brightened and let me know "yes." We went to Kunze Farms again and bought an apple and then drove around for a while. If I listen, I can get the drift of her mood, and she can communicate ideas. I knew she wanted to visit friends, that she likes where she's living. Just pieces of sentences in between mumbling—if strung together, these make an idea.
>
> It angers me that doctors told Dad one and one half years ago that it didn't matter where she was, that she had no awareness. Of course he knew better. She's much worse now, but last week when

Ann and Ken were gone for four days, Mom stopped eating—and started up as soon as they got back. That's communication too! If anyone is paying attention.

And from December 3rd, the same year:

Got to Mom's early (In-service Day) and so took her for a walk. We went around the block twice—she did great. Totally incoherent until we were sitting with Ann and I was telling Ann how Mom had always been a walker and how she lived near the beach in Seattle and walked there every day for thirty years. At this, Mom looked like she was going to cry and said we shouldn't make her remember that.

Finally from December 10th:

Interesting—Ann knew that Mom had a busy day here over Thanksgiving. (We had tromped all over our property, walked up the hill and along the creek.) Mother, although in "severe dementia," can still communicate thought—over time—to anyone paying attention to the mumbling, etc. It does come through. I think she has more thought than words, like a baby. Her thought is impaired but not absent. She still has feelings, reactions, etc., but no longer can use words to effectively express them—unless one is willing to listen over time.

Mrs. Rhodes, The Doctor's cute little roommate and Ken's mother, passed away in November. Mother didn't cry or say anything about it, even when asked, but she didn't want to get out of bed in the mornings, and she wasn't as cheerful until she got a new roommate about nine days later. The new lady, June, was also bedridden and tiny as Mrs. Rhodes had been. We never could tell if The Doctor knew the difference between Mrs. Rhodes and June; she began to tend June immediately, pulling her covers up for her and tucking her in—things that she had always done for Mrs. Rhodes.

One December evening Ralph and I were all dressed up, ready to go to a party when Ann called saying that The Doctor had a temperature of 102 degrees. She had noticed that the last couple of nights Mom had gotten up an extra time in the night to go to the bathroom. Once she had acted as if it hurt. Ann suspected a urinary tract infection. From my journal:

We took her to the Emergency Room at SWWMC [Southwest Washington Medical Center] *... They kept her three hours. It was a bladder infection. They pumped into her one liter of saline solution (to bring the fever down) and antibiotic. They said (1) she was unusually trusting for this kind of patient. I said she has excellent care with no reason to mistrust. (2) They said if I hadn't known the problem (and told them when we came in) it would have been many more hours of tests, etc., to find it. I said Ann knew what it was.*

The Emergency Room nurse said it was unusual also for anyone to know what was wrong with a mentally incompetent patient. I explained that Mom had one-on-one care, like a baby. That's how we knew.

Mom did not appreciate being at the hospital, however:

She was upset when they stuck a catheter in her, not amused when the IV went in, told them to stop when they did the CBC [blood test]. *When they took the tape off her arm to remove the IV, she'd had it and gave me a "Don't-you-tell-me-not-to-be-mad" look and really growled at the nurse!*

In due course she got well, but of course confirming that required a urine specimen. Joy, joy.

The Doctor Agnes, K.E., had loved Dr. Seuss books when we were kids. I can remember her reading them to Tom. One of the benefits of teaching second grade was the fun of reading a Dr. Seuss book aloud. Every year I read *Horton Hears A Who* to my class at the beginning of the year. We would talk about "a person's a person no matter how small." It's an important philosophy to a small person. It was also my way of letting my small students know that they're valued, and that I will hear them when they need to be heard. The same courtesy needs to extend to the mentally incompetent. They are still people, and they have need to be valued and heard.

How can such a simple little philosophy end up being such work? Take Christmas, for example. There was so much of Christmas that The Doctor could still enjoy. She loved going to the Mall and seeing the decorations and lights. Better still were the children waiting to see Santa. She liked going on a drive to look at lights. She went with us to cut a tree, all bundled in her long johns, mittens, and hat. We took her to the children's program at church which featured carols by the congregation. I told friends to greet her as if she was normal and just kind of ignore her mumbling. They did, and it was fine.

I worried over what to do about grandchildren at Christmas, especially those too young to understand how Granny could just forget them. What about lifelong friends far away who could only wonder how The Doctor was doing? Deciding that Mom was a person "no matter how small" meant that she still gave gifts and sent cards. Each remaining year of her life I sent gifts from her to her grandchildren at Christmas and sent Christmas letters, pictures, or cards to her friends. Grandchildren received musical ornaments in 1992. Many of her friends expressed their appreciation to me for letting them know that The Doctor was content, healthy, and loved.

Shortly before Christmas Ann called. From my journal notes:

I want to get each of the ladies something. They have everything they need, though. I think I'll get Belle a doll. She has a fancy doll collection, so I think I'll get her one of those. I don't know what to get your mother." I told her I'd gotten her some slipper socks, a turtleneck, etc. I thought I'd just give her some mittens I have that match her new hat. Ann said, "If I got your mother a fancy doll like Belle's, she'd just take the clothes off of it, and we'd never find them." I said, "How about a baby doll for Mom? She might like that." Ann said, "Well, that's what I was thinking, but I didn't know how you would feel about it. I didn't want to upset you.

So Ann got Mom a doll and called back on Christmas Eve.

She was ecstatic. Mother loves her "new baby." She kisses it and holds it—won't let it out of her sight. Ann said Mom went down the hall saying, "I love you, and I'm going to keep you forever and ever!" I said, "Does she play with it like a child?" Ann said, "No! She's like a mother. She thinks its a real baby. It looks real. This just made my Christmas!"

We decided not to bring The Doctor home overnight that Christmas Eve. She was not comfortable out of her own bed any longer, and was often disoriented if kept away from what had become home for more than about four hours at a stretch. On Christmas Day she did come home with us. Since she and her baby were already inseparable, the baby came home with us too.

By the end of 1992, Mom knew how to get in and out of my car. It had taken over a year, but it interested the teacher in me that she was still capable of learning. After eight months, she called Ann by name.

The Long Goodbye

The last stage of Alzheimer's is sometimes called "the long goodbye." How long? Only God knows. This stage, called Late Dementia, often lasts years. Mother was just beginning this stage about the time she and Dad moved into the Cascade Inn, their retirement apartment. The mood changes and becoming docile were the first real signals that she was going in a new direction. The delusions, mumbling, episodes of incontinence, and eating problems, though slight, were other first steps down a very long road named Goodbye (Gruetzner, 1988).

Chapter 12

1993

Perhaps it wasn't just The Doctor Agnes, K.E., who had gone a little batty. By the first of the year I was buying baby clothes and blankets for our new "family member."

> *Ann says "the baby" has filled a void in Mom's life. It's so weird and beautiful to see her play with it. Weird because it so poignantly points out how far gone she is. Beautiful because she loves it so. She is tender and loving...exactly like a mother with a new baby. She talks to it all the time—incoherently of course, or in Norwegian—possibly both! I told Ann, "You can see why all her children are good talkers!" I asked Ann if Mom ever thought the baby wasn't real. She said, "No, but once your mother noticed there was something wrong with her skin. (The baby is female, Mom decided, and is wearing a scarf—a table napkin I think.) Your mother said, 'She must not be feeling well! Her skin is cold!'"*
>
> *Maybe what is so special about Ann is that she really accepts, enjoys, and loves Mom for who she is right now. Mom feels that. With us "kids" there's sadness, because we know who she was. And Mom feels that, too.*

The Doctor loved her baby completely. Ann felt a little jealous of the doll for a while, because Mom was not as often at her side "helping." I teased her about it. Then my turn came. On a visit one day:

> *Mother—looking at her doll—"I had two baby girls, but they*

weren't as good as this one." Hard to compete.

The baby went on outings with us. Once The Doctor was with me when I got an allergy shot. A lady came up to us and asked me if Mom had Alzheimer's. I said that she did. The woman had cared for her own mother who also had a baby doll. Otherwise people could not tell by looking at her that The Doctor had Alzheimer's. But the baby was a dead giveaway. I sometimes wondered if Dr. Laderas understood the extent of Mom's disability. She asked Mom to tell her my name often when we came in. Mom hadn't known my name since before Dad died. But when I brought Mom in with her baby, there was no mistaking her mental state. It was an eye-opener for Dr. Laderas, actually a good way to help her understand.

The Doctor was very much still out and about. While she hadn't been able to call me by my name for some time, she did know I was family. When I took her out alone, her whole persona became intimate, as if she was with a family member. Even when we couldn't really converse, she seemed to like that feeling of being just with me. Mom was in good shape physically. I took her for frequent walks, as did Ann and Ana (Ann's helper.) Ann also had an exercise machine that The Doctor *loved.* When the weather was wet or cold, Mom exercised indoors. Sometimes I took her to the airport to see Ralph or Heather off. Walking in malls was good exercise too. I often took her on errands with me, usually stopping for a sundae or "split." She came home with me sometimes after work, had dinner with us, and then attended events—especially band concerts—that Janelle was in. She also enjoyed choir concerts at church. Ralph would sit on one side of her, and I on the other. Since she babbled a little, it made some people uncomfortable if they sat right next to her. With Ralph or me between, it was no problem. If I had to ferry Heather around, I could even take The Doctor to Salem with me. She loved going for drives. Still able to read, she would blurt out signs, bumper stickers, or license plates. She also responded to bright colors, especially red. On sharp days she could still identify colors. Most of our trips were short, avoiding the need to use the rest room! She loved driving through well-kept, charming neighborhoods to look at flowers or kids playing. She also enjoyed drives in the country just to see hills, old barns, horses and cows—the same things she'd always enjoyed. I no longer took her inside to eat at restaurants. Her treats were from the drive-through. At one point Ralph and I decided to charge her for all the gas and treats. But that was just a bookkeeping hassle that lasted a few weeks.

Ann also took Mom out with her. She sometimes paid Ana to relieve her only to take The Doctor along! The Doctor was becoming *Ann's* baby! Once Mom and Ann stopped at the Cascade Inn, where Ann left a letter of recommendation from me. Good business. Mom told Connie Easter, the Administrator, that she and Charlie had eaten there! Ann also took The Doctor to garage sales, thrift shops, and all kinds of errands.

It became increasingly difficult to take Mom into a store as the year wore on because of her walk slowing and

> *I have to hold her hand and push the cart at the same time. She can't follow a direction. She can no longer follow me. I finally put her hands on the cart and then pulled the cart from the front—the cart was like a walker for her. This worked well.*

At other times she was difficult because she kept taking things off the shelves or she might try to pull her shirt up or pull her pants down. Taking her into a store became hard work!

Keeping The Doctor Agnes, K.E., attractive for all of these outings was no small thing. She was fighting people who tried to dress her. I explained to Dr. Laderas that if she fought people she might have to be sent to a nursing home—where she would undoubtedly be sedated so she could be managed. Why not sedate her now, so we can leave her where she is? Dr. Laderas agreed. We tried a couple of medications in varying doses, but anything that really helped made her look, feel, and act drugged. Ann loved Mom's personality and decided she would rather have Ana help more and use two people to dress Mom than to have Mom drugged all day. Eventually Ann had to charge us a little more, but that was the best solution to the problem.

At that time, a nursing home or Alzheimer's facility in our area cost between $4,200 and $5,500 per month. In-home care for both Mom and Dad in their Seattle home had cost them $1,500 per month plus board for their live in companion, Sandy. In addition they still had maintenance and normal expenses for their food, other necessities, and home. The Inn had cost about $1,800 per month for the two of them and included food, transportation, activities and entertainment, services like banking, post office, and church. When The Doctor moved into the Assisted Living Wing of the Inn after Dad died, she paid about the same, but got more care. Ann also charged Mom $1,800 when she first moved in. So when Ann upped what Mom was paying by $200 to cover the cost of having Ana help more, we paid $2,000 per month for her. And The Doctor got awesome, one-on-one care.

Tom hosted a garage sale after Dad died. Then he put in some new carpet and had some painting done and so on. John then rented out the house for a time. (We were also looking for a buyer.) Between Mom's social security, the rent from the house, and some interest from a couple of small investments, we could still just about cover the entire cost of what Ann was charging. It was worth spending a little more for Ana to help and for Mom's teeth to be maintained in order to keep her with Ann and out of an institution.

As time went on, The Doctor's glasses also needed replacing. They were so scratched from her abuse. We especially didn't want her to fall for lack of good vision. Ralph asked about having her eyes checked when he went in for glasses, and was assured that they could indeed give The Doctor Agnes, K.E., an exam. We chuckled to ourselves wondering if they'd ever tried with someone like Mom! Still, I made the appointment and took her in. They figured out right away that she couldn't have a regular exam, but Dr. Susan Tenold assured me that they could accurately diagnose what she needed. They could even do it with a newborn! Intrigued, I asked her to explain. She said she would do a retinoscopy with Mom's eyes dilated. All lenses bend light. In a retinoscopy, the ophthalmologist shone a light into the eye. The light bounced back or reflected off the retina in the back of the eye. Dr. Tenold, with her other hand, passed a lens between the light and the eye. She kept doing this, changing lenses over and over, until she found a lens where the light lined up in a straight line. Then Dr. Tenold knew that between Mom's lens in her eye and the lens in Dr. Tenold's hand, the line of vision was correct. She could put a lens with those measurements in

Mom's glasses and have an accurate correction. Magic! We ordered two pairs of glasses, one to wear and one to lose. One set of lenses was installed in Mom's old frames, knowing that the familiarity would help her. Then we ordered another pair in frames as similar to the old ones as we could find. There was no point in getting glasses that she wouldn't wear. When the time came to pick up her new glasses I asked the optician to be especially careful of fit because The Doctor Agnes, K.E., couldn't tell us if it wasn't right. The optician suggested that we watch her carefully. If The Doctor kept taking them off or anything like that, we would need to bring her in again. About a month later we had noticed that she favored one pair—the new one—over the other. I asked Ann to have Mom wear the old pair all day one day, and then I took Mom in the late afternoon back to the optician. Sure enough, the optician found where the glasses made a red spot on Mom, and she was able to adjust them beautifully. She said that Mom might still favor the new ones because they were much lighter to wear.

Another little expense was keeping The Doctor's hair attractive. We were finding it increasingly difficult to take her to the beauty shop to sit for any period of time to have her hair permed. I could trim it a little at Ann's, and we had a hairdresser named Sue Edwards who did a good job with cuts and perms. Sue was willing, but I was having some doubts. Ladies go to hairdressers for a treat, to make themselves look and feel better. I didn't want to hurt Sue's business by having Mom there. Sometimes we made very early appointments to avoid this. I was looking for an alternative way to get Mom's hair done. Heather said she'd give it a try. The experience was so overwhelming that Heather asked if she could write a page in my journal! She wrote:

> *I permed Granny's hair today. It was an adventure. Rolling the hair was no problem; she winced a couple of times if the hair was pulled too tight, but basically sat there with her dolly, clucking to it and kissing it, while I rolled her hair.*
>
> *But she hated it whenever I put her head under any sort of liquid. She couldn't smell the perm solution, of course, but we had no cotton to put around her head, she couldn't think in a straight line long enough to hold a towel or washcloth to her face, and*

hated to get her head wet. It was a chore just to make her bend over to put her head under the faucet, and she wouldn't stay there once liquid was being poured on her head.

The last stage of the perm was the absolute worst, however. After washing out the last of the perm solution, I had to put the neutralizer on and then take it off five minutes later, rinsing for five full minutes. Even getting her to put her head down into the sink was very difficult at this point. She backed away a lot, getting water all over the kitchen. And when I started rinsing her hair, she swore at me: "God damn it, now stop *it!" And she started crying. I tried not to push her or force her much, but as the neutralizer had to come out of her hair, there wasn't a whole lot I could do to "stop it." She was cold and wet by the time we were done. So after I changed her clothes, I sat and rubbed her hands until they were warm. Then I gave her back her baby, and she forgot all about the agony she had just been through.*

My notes from a few days later:

I walked into "Mom's" and there she was, sitting by the fire, rocking her baby—and wearing an Afro! She looked so funny and little with her hair poofed out big all around her head. Fortunately, I came with a comb and hair scissors. First we went for a little drive. I asked her if she wanted to go pick up guys. She said, "Sure." But we just went to the Minit Mart and got gas and a Snickers bar for her. Then we came back, and I gave her a short hair cut—so it would be easy for Ann to keep up. She looks really cute now.

We continued to struggle with hair business. I took her back to Sue a time or two. It wasn't any easier in the shop. Mom could no longer follow a direction, like "lean back." I showed Sue how to give a direction and to physically lean The Doctor back at the same time so that Mom was getting two clues with help *doing* the command. (This was something I had to show hygienists who worked on Mom's teeth also.) If The Doctor wouldn't cooperate, Ann had shown me how to wait a few minutes, doing something else, and then try again. This also worked with dressing her. I showed Sue this, too. Sue was really willing to help. She praised me for keeping Mom's hair up. I told her if all I had left of my self was to look sharp, then I'd better look sharp! Mom deserved the same. Sue also asked about Mom knowing me. I explained: "How little there is left inside of her. She tends to simply reflect what she sees. If people are happy around her, she's happy. If they are sad or worried, she'll be that way. So when I come to see her I always walk in with a big how-nice-to-see-you smile, and so I get the same back from her. It helps both of us. It's a cue for her, a pleasurable response for me."

As I was telling Sue this, Mother picked up a comb and started combing her hair—which Sue had just fixed. Sue said, "Oh, no," and was going to take the comb away but I told her it was OK, that Mom and I were just going out to pick up guys after this, so her hair didn't really matter! Then I pointed out that Mother was doing just what I'd been talking about—reflecting what was around her. She saw Sue combing my hair, so she began to comb her hair. I'm sure that's part of why she "helps" Ann so much. The Doctor sees Ann folding clothes or doing dishes and begins to (try to) do the same thing. The tooth-brushing phenomenon was the same. Ann brushed her teeth, so Mom would brush hers. We both got easy-to-care-for short cuts today. Sue got a big tip. I often tipped Sue $10.00 for a haircut, more for a perm. She was worth it.

The Doctor had a strange thing she did with her hands. Ann said she had seen a former male resident of hers do it also. It looked as if he was sewing. The Doctor would definitely do something in particular with her hands—as if she were making something or fixing something—only the something was not there! We never did figure out what she was doing. It lasted off and on for a short while, perhaps a month. It was a kind of delusion.

One day in early spring, The Doctor and I were on a little walk. She told me that Charlie wasn't making very much money, but that she wasn't worried a bit about it. It was an old tape she was playing that I'd heard her say many times before in earlier years. The truth was that Charlie's money was giving her a comfortable life even years after he was gone. She also would sometimes say that she was dieting, couldn't possibly eat any more. This was another old tape that Ann and I really worried about since she was already so thin!

When I was growing up, Mom always used to say, "You live in your head." She said this if I was upset with someone or discontent about something. It was her way of saying that how you take things, whether you are happy or not, depends upon what is going on in your head. If you're happy there, the rest doesn't matter.

Once I was talking to Janelle about Alzheimer's, about the playing of old tapes, about how hard it was for her to see Granny lose her mind. Janelle said, "I think of the mind as a roomful of file cabinets. In the file cabinets are every memory and thought. Then something comes along and—poof! Starting with the things that just happened and continuing back, it just wipes out the file cabinets one by one."

I said that I thought of it like a tape, and with Alzheimer's the player is broken, so what comes out are bits and pieces. Janelle said the bits and pieces (the things that were so common that bits remain) were cross-referenced in the files all over the place because they were important or long-lived. Then she went on to say that she thought suicide was the choice she'd make if she had Alzheimer's. We talked about the ethics of that for a while, and we talked about how other physical infirmities were different. She held her point, finishing with, "But my mind is where I live."

I said, "Yes, that's what Granny always used to say."

Perhaps that is why I could deal with The Doctor now, though. She was so content. I knew in her head she was happy.

Mother's Day came with the usual wondering from John and Tom about what to send. There were many things The Doctor still enjoyed. I got her a hummingbird feeder because she liked to watch it, wondering if the birds were real. She always liked a corsage because it made her feel dressed up and special for as long as she could wear it. Candy was a favorite. A hanging plant was beautiful for the whole summer; Mom loved fuchsias.

We also got Ann a Mother's Day gift each year—usually a gift certificate for her and Ken to go out for dinner. Ann was such an all-around blessing that we generally gave her something for her birthday and Christmas, too.

By June The Doctor was able to leave pictures on the wall, clothes in her closet, and things in her drawers. Ann was delighted. It made caring for Mom on a minute-to-minute basis a little more relaxed. In truth it meant that Mom was losing the initiative to do things.

Some things remained remarkably intact, though, too. The hospital sent Mom a check in June because between her insurance and me, they had been overpaid for the Emergency Room visit we had made in December. Of course I could have signed for her and deposited it in her account, but I wanted to see if she could still write her name. When I asked her to write her name, nothing except babble happened. When I said, "Write Agnes" she did it. When I said, "Write Leonard" she did that, too. Generally she could no longer follow a direction, but I was finding some exceptions, especially if I caught her just at the right moment.

The Doctor Agnes, K.E., was rapidly losing the use of language. However, she was still able to *communicate*. The last conversations—several sentences strung together in a meaningful way between two or more people—that I can remember with her were at the end of 1991. In 1992 she generally could speak in appropriate sentences, perhaps one or two, in response to someone or something. By 1993 she only rarely spoke in sentences, although she "talked" all the time. Mostly this was in words that did not connect to each other in a meaningful way. Babble. Usually they were in English, but sometimes it was Norwegian. She could still respond with "yes" or "no" to things in a meaningful way. Particularly if a question was asked over and over, one could discern a pattern of similar responses. Often I asked her if she felt good. She might say "sure" one time, "you bet" another, "yes" another. After asking her several times even with much babble in between, I would know that she felt good. She did speak one sentence throughout the year that was meaningful. Each night when Ann tucked her into bed she said, "Thank you for taking such good care of me!"

From the journal in January:

Mom had changed her baby's clothes this week by herself. Ann praised Mom. "Oh, yes, she knew," Ann told me. After some of this, Mother said in a girlish, shy way, "Is it me?" I laughed and said that, yes, it was she who was so good.

This is an example of The Doctor being able to respond in a sentence to others. After one sentence she was "gone" again.

In February I had to pick Heather up in Salem, drive her to Portland's airport, where I would meet Ralph, and leave Heather and her arriving friend with my car. The whole trip took three hours, but it was a beautiful day, so we took Granny along for the ride. All the way to Salem and all the way back, Granny babbled along incoherently. There was not a single thing to come out of her mouth that meant anything at all. When we got to the airport, Heather introduced me to her friend. Then she introduced Granny. Holding her baby in her left hand, The Doctor held out her right hand and said sweetly, "Hello." Heather and I looked at each other and let out a collective sigh of relief!

There were times when Mom was completely coherent and totally inaccurate! Once, when I walked into her home, she was so glad to see me. "Babe!" she said. Turning to Ann, she said, "It's Babe! My sister Babe is here!" I just let her enjoy me as Babe for a while.

She could always communicate a mood. Another day when I came, I knew instantly that she was very angry.

> *She was ticked off today. Ann had been to the doctor and Ana tried to give Mom a shower. No dice. She was still mad when I got there at 4:30. Ann said she'd been agitated all afternoon. She couldn't tell me what was wrong but could answer definitely "yes" or "no" when I asked her questions. "Are you mad today?" "Was someone trying to boss you around?" "Shall we go for a sundae?" She answered "Yes!" to all. The Doctor knew her mind!*

Sometimes I felt that The Doctor could no longer initiate a thought, that now she could only respond. But once when I mentioned Auntie Ethel, she babbled something about Uncle Harold. Associating one thing or person with another *is* a kind of thinking. Other times I felt that she covered up for herself by babbling. If I asked her something she did not know, I sensed from a look in her eye that she *knew* she didn't know, so she just started babbling. The babbling itself seemed intentional, leading me to believe there was thought behind it.

One of the tests done by the U of W asks, in part, for the subject to name common objects. So one day I held up a pencil and asked The Doctor what it was. Nothing. I could get nothing from her remotely responsive to that question. I tried over and over off and on for ten minutes or so. Then finally I handed her the pencil. She immediately began to write with it! So does she know what a pencil is? I'd say so. Did she understand my questions? Probably.

In the summer from the journal:

> *It is no longer possible, generally, to pick up a thread of thought from Mom's ramblings. I can still tell her mood by her tone and the expression on her face. Sometimes she looks at me with such love—the love of a child for its mother; it can be unnerving. Sometimes still she'll be coherent. I took her on a couple of errands. When we went into Parr Lumber to pick up a sack of sand for a little brick patio I am building, the man at the counter said to Mother, "And how are you today?" She said, "Warm!" It was about 95 degrees out! When we got back to Ann's, Ann told me Mom had a scarf this past week and had danced with it kind of like a strip-tease, except she left her clothes on. Ann showed me how Mom had done this and turned around and gave us a wiggle with her rear end—Ann was in shorts—and Mom lit up and said, "I really like that!" She always got a kick out of men and liked things that were just slightly naughty.*

I told Betty about this, and she laughed and said Mom was always lots of fun.

Another day Ann and I were visiting. Ann was upset about someone and telling me all about it when "all this bitching!" popped out of Mom's mouth! She really never swore before Alzheimer's that I could remember.

For Mom's 77th birthday, I took her for a little tourist train ride to a beautiful forested waterfall. As luck would have it there was an old guy on the train who was paying some attention to her, but she wasn't interested. She didn't like the bumpy train ride, although she enjoyed the waterfall and forest. Homer and Betty came a few days later for a little luncheon at my house. The Doctor even danced with Homer when I put some jazzy music on.

Mom continued to journey back in time. She asked for Charlie less and less, her parents, brothers, and sister more and more. She only rarely asked about Babe, perhaps because Babe was a few years younger than Mom and Mom—in her own head—was only a few years old. The Doctor's actions were very girlish—the way she looked and laughed and moved—even the look in her eyes. She was not nearly as interested in flirting with men. Ann and I decided together not to keep telling her that so much of her family had passed away. It only made her sad. Instead we would tell her that they were fine, they loved her, she would see them soon.

Paradoxically, The Doctor thought about dying from time to time. One day in February on a long drive:

> *Somewhere inside her she is thinking of dying. She thought a church was a mortuary when we drove around as she ate her hot caramel sundae with nuts. She mentioned Yarrington's Funeral Home in Seattle where she once worked. She asked me where I wanted to be buried. She asked twice how Dad died. And when. She was coherent for a few sentences today. These bits and pieces came out over a period of two hours. They were totally engulfed in babble. Still, if one* listens, *the thread of thought comes through.*

I also thought about The Doctor dying, kind of planning her funeral in my head. Sometimes it seemed as if she couldn't possibly keep going like this, helpless and frail. At other times it looked as she would go on for years. Her weight stabilized in 1993; Mom lost only five pounds in the course of the whole year, although she still had a few bouts of an upset stomach, but very few. In addition she had taken to playing with her food:

> *Mom was playing with her food when I arrived. She'd put cookies in her soup, soup on her bananas and so on ...*

Ann was feeding her at least one meal per day because of this. At other times The Doctor would eat just fine by herself. (Ann didn't ever let The

Doctor skip meals.) Once when Ken and Ann went on a trip to Mexico, Ann's sister Hazel came and took over. Hazel does this kind of work in Oklahoma. Another sister took over for *her*! Anyway, Hazel came up with the idea of giving The Doctor chewable children's vitamins. Mom liked that much better than trying to take a pill. Meanwhile Ann had figured out that Mom liked her pills best in a spoon of ice cream. Ann also would leave food out for The Doctor. She might leave out a banana or muffin, even a chewable vitamin. What The Doctor wouldn't eat one minute, she might eat the next.

It was even more remarkable that Mom's weight stabilized, considering that she had a long series of bladder infections. She had a few episodes of daytime incontinence one week in early February. By the next week, Ann was suspecting a bladder infection because The Doctor had gotten up two extra times in the night to go potty. I took her in and of course this required my favorite procedure, the urine specimen. Sure enough, it was another bladder infection. Best of all, could we come back a week or so after the medication was finished for a re-check?

I was relating long-distance the joys of medical procedures one day to my sister-in-law, Marilyn, who has experience as a geriatric nurse. She suggested a device called a hat to collect urine. It fits between the toilet and the toilet seat and collects the urine. I could collect the urine at Ann's before I took Mom in. Refrigerated for a short time in a sterile jar, it would still be usable for Dr. Laderas. I asked where I might get such a hat. Marilyn explained that there are drug stores and other such places that specialize in all manner of medical devices and equipment. I found a place that did indeed have a hat. Cost: $2.50. I probably would have been willing to spend about a hundred times that much for this device! Not only did the hat work, but I had found an outfit that would help me with all kinds of future problems, large and small. It took me another year to figure out that Health Tek Pharmacy would even *deliver* everything from diapers to prescriptions, putting them on my Visa.

For a while daytime incontinence was a signal to us of a bladder infection. The Doctor had bladder infections again in May, July, September, October, and November. By the end of the year Mom was incontinent much of the time, so we could no longer use this as a clue. Again we looked at the ethics of the whole situation. Was it right to pray for the good Lord to take her and then keep treating chronic infections? Each time the infection would be totally gone after a course of antibiotics, only to come back again. Sometimes, these are not treated in older people. Once again, I was glad not to be in this alone. John, Tom, and I decided to ask Dr. Laderas if we should stop treating the infections unless Mom was in pain. Dr. Laderas agreed.

One very odd thing happened to Mom on a certain medication for her bladder infections. After the first few infections, Dr. Laderas tried a relatively new, fairly potent drug called Maxaquin. Each time Mom was on Maxaquin she became markedly more coherent! One October journal entry:

I saw Mom yesterday. She was more coherent than she has been in several months—which is to say she said several coherent sentences over the course of 45 minutes or so. She pointed out Ann to me and told me how pretty and how good she is and how much she just loves her. I looked through a photo album I made for her some time ago with snapshots of her S. Dakota days and trips all over the world, and of good friends and family. I showed her a picture of Dad and asked, "Who is that?" She said, "Charlie!" At one point she said, "They all died before I died, didn't they?" I was so shocked. I said, "But you haven't died!"

[Concerning a new drug that can help Alzheimer's victims in the early stages of the disease, I had been wondering how I would feel if they ever found something for The Doctor.] *It's rather uncanny, unsettling when she has these brief moments of knowing. It's almost harder to see this than when she's just "gone." There's something horrifying in the thought of her "coming back." Earlier she was horrified at losing her mind. She knew it was happening. I wouldn't want to bring that back for her, even if she would be more coherent, unless the degeneration of the disease was also gone, unless she was completely cured. Why go through losing your mind twice? With very limited ability to really think, she now lacks the capacity to be horrified any more. She also told Ann today that she was an old woman with nothing rattling around in her head. Even at her best she is coherent for just a sentence or two, a short moment. She even laughed at a little joke I made today. I wonder if it is because she's at the end of her course of antibiotics for bladder infections. She is feeling especially well. Ken told me last week how much he admired how I could relate to Mom. I thought afterwards that it takes two people to "relate"; there's only one of us "home!" But today, I connected with the other for the first time in a very long time. I looked into her eyes when she laughed at the joke and saw Mother in there looking out at me, and I knew she got it, and she knew I knew. I could see that she was feeling triumphant about it. Somehow this was so hard for me to take. I'm getting a little nutty over this anyway. I've even thought recently how freeing death will be for her. I want to see her break free of the chains of that tangled mind. Mother once loved to think and outsmart someone. She was a reader and forever curious. Once on the beach when I was a kid she saw a geoduck's neck sticking out of the sand. A kind of clam, they were so fast, so hard to dig for. She said, "I wonder what would happen if I just grabbed his neck?" Quick as lightning, she did! And then stood screaming on the beach because she was standing there with just a geoduck's neck in her hands! Curiosity killed the cat. She went to college even though her mother told her she didn't need an education. She was proud of her mind. I saw that in her for a second or two today.*

A few weeks later:

It took me a while to be able to articulate this: What upset me when Mom was more coherent—when I could look her in the eye and there she was—was the horror of seeing, "My God, she's still in there!" Trapped in that body. She is still there. Not totally "gone." Once in a while she can still peek out and see the world as it is.

The next month (November) Hazel was again taking care of things.

Ken and Ann were in Colorado. After another round of Maxaquin, The Doctor Agnes, K.E., needed no help getting in and out of my car—for the first time in about a year. Also:

> She had a picture of herself and Dad. I said, "Who's that?" She said, "That's my baby." I said, "He's pretty handsome, isn't he?" She said, "Charlie?" I nodded. She said, "Yes, he is." I said to Hazel, "When you first came two weeks ago you were shocked at how much Mom had declined just since July. Do you still think she's so bad?" "Oh no," she said.

It had been nearly *two years* since I had that much of a conversation with The Doctor. From my journal:

> *Meredith* [Pfanschmidt, the RN in charge of the Alzheimer's study that Mom is in at the University of Washington] *called me at work yesterday and said she was forwarding my "interesting reports" to a physician. I sure hope somebody will pay attention to this, because it's* unreal!
> *The Maxaquin effect will wear off again soon.*

Homer and Betty visited before it wore off though, and Mother mentioned Harlan, Homer's brother, and Louise, Harlan's wife. It was one thing for The Doctor to talk about very close friends and relatives, but this was something else!

I couldn't talk Dr. Laderas into prescribing Maxaquin for Mom when she was well just to see what it would do...

With increasing incontinence came the need for diapers. Getting Mom in diapers and keeping her there proved to be something of a trial. She would take off her diaper at night, then wet the bed. Then she would go into the other bed in her room, go to sleep in it, and wet it, too! It was as if mentally she was in one place while physically she was in another. Once The Doctor pooped in the waste paper basket—in spite of the bathroom all lit up right there. (Mom's room was the master bedroom of the house.) Another time she pooped on a pillow and then very neatly placed it in a corner of the room where Ana discovered it in the morning! Mercifully, this stage was short.

By about the middle of the year, The Doctor also needed help going to the bathroom during the day. She needed help finding the toilet, taking down her pants, and so on. After she peed on Ann's floor one day, I worried to Ann about her floors and carpets, but she said she had a $300.00 machine that took care of it just fine. (The woman is an angel.) Ann's home was always immaculately clean. Although The Doctor was in diapers round the clock by the end of the year, it was still possible for her to use the toilet most of the time by keeping her on a regular bathroom schedule and by watching her. This continued for *years*. She had a couple of what we first thought were diaper rashes, but Dr. Laderas said they were external yeast infections—probably from the antibiotics—and gave us a prescription for a cream that cleared them right up.

Several changes occurred in the autumn. Mom's moods became less upbeat. She would cry more, again child-like. When I took her for a flu shot, she had to be held tight, because she just could not understand why someone would hurt her. Perhaps these changes were related to the recurring bladder infections. I think she felt well only off and on that fall and early winter. Sometimes she would be curled up in her bed in a fetal position. Often she was stuporous, unresponsive to others in the room. I found myself visiting more frequently. We wondered if we were losing her.

When Thanksgiving came around, we had company from all over. Heather brought her Japanese roommate and her fiancé from Florida. We decided not to bring Mom home for the feast. Ann had a Thanksgiving dinner at her place and said it was just as well if The Doctor stayed there.

We did bring The Doctor home for Christmas, though. She walked to the creek with me, laughed delightedly when she saw it, and said, "Oh" and gestured with her hands at how lovely the creek was. The creek and my home were new to Mom each time she came. Each time she enjoyed the serenity and natural beauty as if for the first time.

...We had gotten a new dog, and it was a beautiful day, so we all spent some time on the deck with the dog. Mom seemed to really be enjoying the liveliness of it all.

Yes, she could still communicate.

We had done other Christmas things with her, too. She had seen decorative lights and heard carols at church. Cards with pictures were sent to her friends for her, and she received pictures and notes from old and dear friends and relatives. She loved looking at those things; they seemed to take her back even further in time.

Chapter 13

Meanwhile

While The Doctor Agnes, K.E., was lost in the space of late dementia, there was a lot going on around her that she missed, but that had bearing on her care and on those who cared for her.

My own family entered an extremely busy time. Heather, who was a student in international relations and mathematics at Willamette University in Salem, Oregon, spent a semester in France in 1992. After returning home, she met a young man over the Internet. Marc McConley was a grad student at M.I.T. Thus began a coast-to-coast romance. They were engaged in 1993, the year Heather graduated, and married in 1994. As a practical matter, it meant that while we were caring for Granny, we were back and forth some with Heather in college, and we went through wedding preparations! Throughout Heather's college career, she lived with students from Japan. These students were guests in our home for holidays and breaks. Heather worked summers and vacations for a temporary employment service that kept her busy full-time. In the summer of 1993 she went to Alaska and did "hard time" in a cannery.

Janelle was in high school with a full schedule there. She stage-managed six plays, though her friends said it was actually stage-*mangling*. When rehearsals went late, as they often did, I would take my turn stopping after work at fast food and grocery stores to get dinner for the cast and crew. It was a fun diversion for me. I'd walk in loaded with burgers, chips, Coke, and—for my conscience—fruit. The kids would come running up to me saying things like, "Oh, Mother Akin, may I kiss your feet?!" This had the desired effect of prompting return visits. It was a fun group, and I knew them well, not only from plays, but from parties and other visits at our home. Janelle was also involved in band. She played French horn in the symphonic and marching bands, keyboard in the pep band, and piano in the jazz band. She played in concerts, parades, contests, and games. In addition, she belonged to a group called Natural Helpers, did some fund-raising for National Honor Society, and was just a busy girl all around. When wedding preparations for Heather began, Janelle arranged all of the music for it and took the musicians through rehearsals. Janelle worked summers at a horse camp called Royal Ridges. She had started as a camper in fifth grade, and so it was a place that really captured her heart. By the end of her senior year, though, she worked both in fast food and for a temporary employment service.

A major event in Janelle's senior year was getting her tonsils out. She was wheeled into surgery singing "I'm Too Sexy For My Shirt," a reference to her hospital gown, but she didn't sing much for about a week after.

Then Janelle went off to college at the University of Rochester in New York, after graduating from high school in 1994.

Ralph and I were just gasping for breath amid all of the activity. Between our jobs, kids, church, Rotary for Ralph, graduations, a wedding, and The Doctor, we simply tried to survive. Volunteering in a variety of capacities had always been part of our lives. We volunteered in things related to our church, community, family, and jobs. We always worked alongside interesting people, and it was a good way to gain a wider and healthier perspective of many things—including ourselves. During this time, however, our volunteer activities slowed to a minimum. I would sometimes ask Mr. Bruner, the drama coach, if he needed any help when I stopped by with dinner for everyone. I might get sent on an errand to pick up a prop or something. I also rocked babies in the nursery at church on a regular basis. Both Ralph and I did a little assisting with Sunday School classes at church. We took our turns at interstate rest stops making coffee and offering cookies—part of band fund-raising. However, I was not into organizing, managing, or being chairperson of any great things just then. This wasn't the time for it. Ralph, although he stayed quite busy with Rotary and worked on an exchange with Russian students coming to the United States, was less involved than he had been. It was one area where we could cut back.

Ken once told me that he admired how I handled Mom, saying that being uncomfortable and wanting to keep at a distance was more common. I'm not sure I handled it *better* than others, just differently. Besides going through menopause at this same time, I developed all kinds of allergies and asthma. Not particularly admirable in my mind.

I needed to talk about The Doctor, to mentally work through some of the issues I was trying to handle:

I fear that I bore people about Mother. I try not to. Ralph is patient and listens. He knows I need to talk it out. Sue—where I get my hair done—wants to hear about it. A couple of colleagues ask regularly. I talk to John and Tom, my aunts, Homer and Betty. My feelings about growing old have changed. Long life doesn't seem a worthy goal...between taking care of Mom, my allergies, and menopause, I'm a tad neurotic about my health. If I got Alzheimer's, I wouldn't want to move in with my children.

Between Mom and Janelle and ten days of overnight company last month, I'm glad my class is peachy. I feel like I haven't had a moment to breathe since school started. I worked till 7:30 on Thursday this week. Got home at 7:00 on Friday, having seen Mom. Ralph and I went hot-tubbing. Today—at last—a real day off. Heather was home last weekend; the weekend before we had company. I do feel the weight of holding up both generations—I'm sure Ralph does, too.

I'm ready to lose Mom now, though she might hang on for some time yet. Had she died right after Dad died, I would have felt guilty. Now I'm ready—partly because I'm tired; I want to get on with my life. Partly I'd like to have time with Janelle before she leaves home for college next fall, unencumbered by Mom. And partly I want it now for Mom. She needs to be free. I'm going for a walk.

I didn't always work late, of course. If Mom needed to see a dentist, or Janelle had something going on, I could leave as early as 4:00 P.M. However, when Ralph was out of town and Janelle was busy with rehearsals, I could and did stay late to really dig in at school.

I also began to do things just for me. We bought a hot tub that both girls and their friends thoroughly enjoyed, but we bought it as a treat for Ralph and me. In the spring of 1993, I went to Phoenix to visit with Auntie Ethel, and the two of us took a trip to the Grand Canyon.

Ralph and I went to Alaska that year to visit his sister's family in Juneau and Tom's family in Anchorage. John had asked me if we were going to go to Glacier Bay from Juneau also, since I had mentioned before that I really wanted to do that. I told him I didn't think we could afford it this time, what with a wedding coming and college costs. He said, "What if I paid for it?" What a generous offer! However, I said, no, that wasn't necessary. Then I thought, "But I would let the estate pay for it." He said to do it. This was an acknowledgment of all we had done for The Doctor. It was still very generous. So Ralph and I flew in a small plane right *through* the coastal Alaskan mountains to Glacier Bay where we spent a glorious long day on a boat cruising, watching whales and other wildlife, and viewing glaciers, compliments of The Doctor. A week later with Tom we caught enough salmon and halibut to last a whole year. I caught a 68-pound king salmon on the Kenai River! Tom and Teri really treated us to a fabulous time.

Homer and Betty continued to stop by to see Mom regularly every few months. As The Doctor generally deteriorated at the end of 1993, I kept them current. They, in turn, kept other Seattle friends apprised of how The Doctor was doing. Mabel Patterson, Mom's dear friend from South Dakota days, continued to send Mom notes and pictures several times a year. Mabel had a stroke a few years earlier and lived with one of her children, so she wasn't able to come down.

Ann had told me when I first moved Mother in with her that her home was like a family, that even relatives of residents became like family. I hadn't given it much thought at the time, but those words came back to me often. The longer Mom was there, the more I could see that it was true.

When Belle passed away in January 1993, she had been with Ann for nearly three years. Ann kept her until the night before she died. Belle complained of some abdominal pain that night—for the first time—and Ann called her family and suggested that they take her to the Emergency Room.

Belle was gone by morning. Ann grieved for Belle, vowing to never get so close to one of her residents again. It did no good. Ann loved her people and that was what made her home so special. It was her nature to love. Already she was very attached to The Doctor.

In the spring Mom's roommate, June, wasn't doing well. Then it looked as if she was better, and Ken and Ann decided to use the opportunity to take a quick weekend camping trip. Ann had a young woman, Sunshine, who sometimes worked for her. Sunshine came for the weekend with a friend to care for the ladies, with Ana from across the street also checking in. Alas, poor June passed away quietly in her sleep that weekend. Sunshine called me, asking me to come and take The Doctor for a little while because she was worried that all the people in and out might bother Mom. This was not something Ann would ever have done, but I knew Sunshine and was glad to do anything to help her. Although she was trained and licensed, she was young, and this had upset her. So I went over. She had everything nicely under control. I asked if she needed anything else and then took Mom with me for a few hours.

For a little while Ann had only one or two residents. This is when she was taking Mom on errands with her. Ann also took Mom to her own hairdresser a time or two. I could just give Ann a signed blank check to get Mom's hair done. It really was like a family. Ann even took a urine specimen to Dr. Laderas for me once. She was doing *my* errands!

When I went to visit I knocked twice and walked in. I would help myself to a glass of water or a cup of coffee. If I made jam, I'd take over a jar of it. Ann's specialty was cinnamon rolls, and she sent some home with me. This is the kind of give-and-take that occurs in a family or between very close friends. It was such a *comfortable, positive* way to be able to visit Mom, not at all like visiting her in an institution.

Some journal notes:

> *Mom was just finishing her dinner—homemade beef stew, a salad, a bowl of cottage cheese. She ate only the salad completely. Heather and I stopped in a couple of days ago, too, and Heather borrowed a jacket from Mom for her trip to Florida to meet Marc's family. Mom wasn't there then—Ann had taken her out*

shopping to a fabric or craft store!

I ran errands and worked at school all day. Then I stopped in to see Mom. She was sitting in the living room babbling away. Ann and her bookkeeper were in the dining room going over the books. So Mom and I took off for K-Mart where I needed to pick up some fertilizer and Deadline to get rid of slugs in my garden...Ann said she [Mom] needed bras and socks. I ordered two bras because her others are way too big now and some bright slouch socks for her from the Penny's catalogue.

Ann had tried someone else's bra on Mom, and was able to tell me what size to get from that. This sounds like a small thing, but taking The Doctor to a department store to try on bras would have been a major undertaking—and not a pleasant one! This is the kind of service that would never have come from any kind of institutional care.

I had to appear in court this morning to testify about our creek running mud last winter. I had a sub for the morning. Since I was finished at 10:00 A.M. I stopped in to see Mom...Ann wasn't there today, she had run to the store, so conversation at the breakfast table was interesting. There was Mom—totally gone—and Ana who doesn't speak much English—and Mom's new roommate who is kind of in and out...still, it beat sitting nervously in court!

Not everyone fit into Ann's eclectic foster home. Not everyone who came became part of this family. Ann went to great lengths to help new residents do well there. When June first came she was angry, unhappy, and had a backside full of bedsores. Within a week she was loving and grateful. Her bedsores eventually disappeared. Ann took pride in making sure even her bedridden patients got excellent care. Not everyone could pay the full price. Medicaid paid only about $1,100 per resident. Ann would take one of these at a time, even though that hardly covered expenses. It was charitable for her to do that. Sometimes an extended family would pay some of the difference between what Medicaid paid and what Ann charged. Several people came to Annabelle's Foster Care who didn't try to fit in, for a variety of reasons. Sometimes health problems were too severe. Sometimes a resident would intentionally upset others to get attention or even to get "kicked out," because they hoped to go to their own homes again. Sometimes a family did not cooperate in the care. If a patient needed medication, and the family did not take the patient to the doctor, Ann did not want to be held responsible. If a resident was not working out, after a while Ann would ask their families to find another place for them. Sometimes the personalities simply did not mesh.

Notes from the journal:

There's a new lady this week—a stroke victim—very spoiled, Ann says. I can't imagine that anyone is more spoiled than what Ann gives toward her people. But some of these folks rule their families, lay on the guilt, want to be in their own homes, etc. And sometimes it only lands them in a nursing home. They'd be smarter to know a good thing when they see it.

Ann's new lady didn't last long. She wanted Ann to sit and talk to her all night long each night and when Ann wouldn't, she cussed her out. Also did her little cussing fits when her husband would come to visit—so he'd take her home. So he did, and she felt so smart about it. The sad thing is she needs care, hubby is a merchant marine, leaving again next week, and her daughter says there's no way she'll take her mother. The woman probably outsmarted everyone so well she'll land in a nursing home under sedation. Brilliant.

The new lady, Ellen [this is a different woman who had some of her care paid for by the state and some by her family] *has a niece who was late paying Ellen's share. Ann can be tough about her business. I don't mind paying well and on time and giving Ann little bonus gift certificates from time to time. We're getting wonderful care out of the deal.* [I had overheard Ann on the phone with the niece.]

[Months later] *Ellen is such a sweet roommate. She helps Mom, I think. Mom's always getting into her things—and her bed! I think she just enjoys the company though.*

Ellen moved out. She needs hip surgery and then therapy so will be in a nursing home for a while. Ann was going to let her come back, but when they left they put two holes in the wall about two inches in diameter each—right through the wallpaper. When Ann called Ellen's family about it, they said in effect, "Well, tough luck." Ann could take them to small claims court for the cost of repair and new wallpaper but probably won't. She also won't have Ellen back either. I feel bad for Ellen.

Yesterday Ralph took Mom in for her quarterly teeth cleaning. Janelle had a tonsillectomy last week, and I had taken time off for that—as had Ralph—so it just worked out that he took Mom to the dentist. When they returned, they just walked right in as usual— Ann and Ken are like family now and their place like home. There was a new lady sitting in the dining room looking at a book. Since Ralph didn't see Ann, he went to the door of their apartment adjoining the dining room and [standing next to the lady] knocked a couple of times. The new lady looked up and said, "Would you like me to get that?" Ralph is only rarely left speechless.

This was our introduction to Nina, who also suffered from Alzheimer's. I also got attached to the residents. Nina was a bit gruff and rough, lacking tact. She reminded me some of Mom a few years earlier. What I loved most about her was a wonderful, dry sense of humor accompanied by the cutest twinkle in her eye. Nina also came with a son and daughter-in-law. The daughter-in-law, Bonnie, solved our hair problems for quite some time. She was a hairdresser and would come and do the ladies' hair right at Ann's.

Residents came and went. Some left because they needed therapy or round-the-clock skilled nursing care. Some left because they or their families were a problem. Some passed away. The Doctor sailed right through the changes, not noticing many of them.

Even though The Doctor was in a place that was long-term and homey now, John and Tom agonized over coming to see her.

John and Tom ask me if they should see Mom. I never know

what to say. I say it makes no difference to her now. Really it doesn't. I say if they need to see her a last time, then come. I talked to Ken about it because he went through this with his mom. He pointed out the blessing and benefit of being able to remember Mom as she was. Even she would want to be remembered that way. I can hardly remember her the way she was anymore—until a rare moment comes along, and then I see her.

It was very difficult for John to see Mom. It tore him up. I felt that he should see her only if he felt he needed to. John did many other things to show his love for Mom. He took care of all of her finances. He supported me. Any time I needed to buy something for Mom, I had his blessing. He always told me to spend whatever it took to keep her comfortable and happy. He never questioned my care of her, whether it was trips to the doctor, dentist, hairdresser, or the whole new wardrobe I had gotten for The Doctor. However, seeing Mom was difficult for John. I know he felt guilty about not coming often. I told him what Ken had said, that Mom would appreciate him remembering her as she was without Alzheimer's.

John was also a completely honest sounding board. Where Tom and I might see things one way, I could count on John to look at them from a different angle and give me his slant on it. He pulled no punches:

John called. The house still hasn't sold. We may have to drop the price again. John may go over and sell it himself, enabling him to drop the price. He has my support whichever way it goes.

I filled him in on all Mom's news. [This was in the fall when she wasn't doing well because of recurring bladder infections.] *He said maybe I shouldn't get Mom a flu shot this year; anything even potentially to prolong her life could be cruel. He said there's no dignity for someone who wets their pants, poops on the floor, etc. If she could step back to who she was and see who she is now, it would be appalling, shocking. All of what John said has truth. I need to re-think things again. Just when I've mentally decided what I'll do if this happens or that happens, something new comes along for me to think through. Of course John said he'd support anything I do either way; it's my call.*

Ralph said if we knew Mom would get the flu and be gone in three days, it would be an easy decision. However, she could also be sick for two months, infect others, and get well—which sounds a lot like Mom's health.

Ann has a new resident—a new roommate for Mom. Her name is Christine, and she has had a stroke, so she cannot speak. She can' make noises and smile, though. She's incontinent, too. Ann says Christine's daughter comes over and cries when she sees Christine. She says Mom just reaches over and pats Christine when Christine tries to talk. Ann says Mother will have dignity to the very end—because she can still reach out in love to another human being.

Tom had less trouble seeing Mom. He could accept and love her as she was without hurting the way John did.

Babe and Larry made a trip up from Texas in the fall of 1993. They spent the better part of a day with The Doctor who was in sharp form. She even called Larry by name once! They could see that Mom was loved and beautifully cared for. It saddened Babe especially to see her sister. She felt glad that she had come but was also glad to leave. Later she once mused that perhaps she shouldn't have come.

I didn't have the luxury of being able to walk away from The Doctor. I did, however, have the blessing of visiting her in a loving home. I might find her under a big umbrella having lunch with the other ladies by summer, out in the yard in fall or spring picking flowers, or rocking her baby by the fire in the winter. Mom was happily oblivious to the effects her life was having on everyone else.

Chapter 14

1994

1-1-94. Sweet Christine got pneumonia before Christmas and went to the hospital where she had another stroke. They had to put tubes in her to feed her, so she had to go to a nursing home. That's a hard call to make, too—particularly since with Christine being a stroke victim, there is a possibility of getting better. To me that is a critical difference. We can fix Mom's bladder—maybe—but she won't ever get better. I won't put tubes into her. But I miss Christine and her clicking communication—and she was getting better. Her speech was returning, and I had praised her for it.

1-21-94. I went to see mom after work. She was much better today. I took her on a little drive, and we stopped at a new Pier One Import store. She still likes to see lovely things. We walked a little; it was a beautiful evening, fairly warm. Mom got in and out of my car today with no help at all. Ann said she even danced some today and Ken told me that when he got home, Mom greeted him with open arms! I said, "That must make you feel really welcome around here!" Ken has to be some kind of saint to live with all the extra people in his home.

I have been wanting to make a tape recording of mom for a long time. Of course at the beginning of Alzheimer's she just repeated herself, asking the same questions over and over or having the same conversations time and again. Then she got so that, while she was still coherent, she was just wrong. Once she told Ann she had been married twice, for example, when she has only been married once. Now she is only rarely coherent. Often she mumbles in nonsense syllables that aren't even words. I taped a "conversation" with her today because she was far more coherent than I have heard her in the last few months. Still, it's not much:

C: *How are you feeling today?*
A: *Fine. I haven't got anything with (mumble)*
    (Laughter from both)
C: *What have you been up to today?*
A: *I have absolutely been zilch.*
C: *Zilch?*
A: *Because they got two and they got one, huh?*
C: *Who?*
A: *Lunch. They and Mrs. Lunch*
C: *Mrs. Lunch?*
A: *Agnes.*
C: *Agnes? That's your name?*
A: *Well, I'll teaching school and I and I want to go back to that?*
    [She has identified herself here as a teacher and is asking if she
    can go back to that.]
C: *Yeah.*
A: *I hate...they took the neatest down (pause) and back. (Swoosh*
    sounds with big gesture) I don't—why I'm in for good with
    these people. Me but you could just some (mumble) I. They
    could. [I think here she is referring to her living situation. She
    may be upset with someone, perhaps Ann for moving things
    around following Christine's departure.]
C: *They could?*
A: *Yeah. There they go (mumble)*
C: *How are you feeling today?* [I often repeat questions because
    with repetition I can get an idea from several responses. A
    pattern will emerge. Generally I ask her several times each
    time I see her how she is feeling. If I think there might be pain,
    I ask about that repeatedly also.]
A: *(Positive sounds) Fine.*

C: *You look like you feel better than you were the last time I saw you.*

A: *Yeah?*

C: *Yeah. Are you cold?*

A: *(laughs)*

C: *Are you cold?*

A: *No, I don't want to get up into the light.*

C: *You don't want to get up into the light—but you're not cold are you?*

A: *Look for direction...*

C: *No.*

A: *(mumble)*

C: *What do you think of that new big-screen TV?*

A: *Oh? Does that mean (mumble)......Charlotte and Ralph.*

C: *Charlotte and Ralph. Who're Charlotte and Ralph?*

A: *Well, (mumble)*

C: *Who am I?*

A: *I haven't seen before and I saw it though one day when I tried and they peach—peaches rows until I tried to sound different. (clears her throat, mumbles)*

C: *Where's your baby today?*

A: *(Mumble)*

C: *What're you doing?*

A: *You have got something (mumble)*

C: *What have you been doing today?*

A: *Oh today (mumble) Is a cat outside (points out the window) Looks good for us*

C: *I don't see a cat. Can you see a cat out there?*

A: *Mumble*

C: *I can't either.*

A: *No (mumble) do is for d for d*

C: *Do you know what I'm doing?*

A: *Yeah.*

C: *Here, sit down and I'll tell you what I'm doing. I'm making a tape recording of you talking.*

A: I'm much better if I could get just get two.

C: Oh I think you're gonna sound just fine.

A: Yeah (with feeling!)

C: I think it will be interesting to have a tape recording. Don't you think?

A: Do you think we'll have to walk home? [Of course we were "home."]

C: Well, I don't think we'll have to walk home (in a comforting tone).

   Would you like to go for a little drive?

A: And what's it.

C: It's a nice afternoon. Would you like to go for a drive?

A: I don't think I'm can hardly (mumble) going to talk to these kids about this.

C: You're going to talk to these kids about these things? Would you like to go for a ride? Let's go for a ride in the car, shall we?

A: Should she (mumble) See I don't have at all (mumble) [Then she got up and went over to the closet and opened the door, which I took as my cue that she wanted to go for a ride, so I took her out of the little bedroom we were in and we went down the hall to another closet where her coat was. Then I bundled her up and we went out.]

Mother was declining steadily at the end of 1993 with a series of bladder infections that were becoming chronic. She also had some general itching—particularly when she wasn't eating well. Her appetite ran hot and cold, her urine was cloudy, and her disposition was touchier. I wondered if her kidneys were slowly shutting down. Early in January at the end of one visit, Ann was guiding The Doctor back to her room when Mom jumped as if in pain. I asked Ann if this was new. Ann said she had only done it once before, earlier in the same day. The Doctor, like an infant, was not able to tell us why she hurt, or where. Indeed there had been times when she *should* have hurt but did not. Her pain threshold seemed to be rising. Dick Moller, her dentist, had commented when the long work on her teeth and gums was being done that it was amazing that she hadn't been in pain with it. In fact it wasn't until well after her teeth were completely fixed that she began losing weight. So we knew that infected gums, loose dental plates, abscesses, and decay hadn't bothered her at all. Now, however, she was feeling pain. I gently pushed on her lower back and abdomen. There was definite pain and tenderness on one side, both front and back, just below her waist. I could watch her face as I prodded here and there to tell where the pain was. She would wince. We made an appointment for her to see the doctor.

Ann gave Mother some medicine before I took her to the doctor the next day to help calm her. Experience said she would not be amused by having to get out of her clothes only to get poked and prodded. Ann also had a urine specimen ready to go. However, by the time we got to see Dr. Laderas in the late afternoon, the pain was gone. Dr. Laderas did a couple of other tests, including a blood test, but everything came out fine. (One kidney reading that refers to the filtering function of the kidneys came out high. Dr. Laderas said that since other clinical indications were normal, this generally just meant that she might be slightly dehydrated.) This time there was no sign of infection. Ralph suggested that evening that perhaps The Doctor Agnes, K.E., had passed a small kidney stone. This would explain both the pain and its disappearance. I thought nothing of it for some time. But when several months had passed without another bladder infection, it seemed more probable that there might have been an obstruction in her urinary tract that caused infection and later pain when she passed it. We never knew for sure, though.

Mom's weight for most of her adult life was around 140 pounds. She was five feet six inches tall with a medium to large frame, so she was just about right—not surprising, given her love of exercise and the number of diets she tried on both herself and Dad. At the the Cascade Inn they weighed her regularly, and when she left she weighed 145 pounds, fully dressed with shoes. In January of 1994 The Doctor weighed just 104 pounds, again fully dressed. By March she weighed 98 pounds. I was thinking about taking her to Heather's wedding or perhaps just the reception, but she could just about swim in all of her better dresses. I went out and bought her a new pink suit, size six.

It fits perfectly. She looks so little and thin. It's always shocking to me to see her without clothes. Even her chest is bony. But I found a dusty pink suit with pleated skirt in a crepe. It's very pretty on her.

Even though the bladder infections were gone, we had other problems besides Mom's weight. In February The Doctor got a case of the flu, in spite of her shot, and I had my first and only disagreement with Ann:

2-24-94. Mom was feverish when I stopped by today. They've all got a chest cold. This is the first time Mom has been sick like this since the spring of '91. We'll see how she does with it. Her temp was 100.2 and she was babbling—the sounds weren't recognizable words in any *language.*

I have to drive Janelle to Seattle tomorrow for a college interview and audition. I'll be back by Sat. afternoon. I'll have Mom's SS card and Medicare card here for Ralph in case of emergency.

2-25-94. As I was getting ready to go to Seattle I called Ann to check on Mom. She had called Dr. Laderas and gotten a Rx from her for some penicillin for Mom, because she was worried about the fever and Mom being so frail. I wasn't comfortable with that from a couple of different angles, so I told Ann to hold off on giving it to her. I asked Ann if Mom was acting any differently from the way the others with the flu were acting. She said no. So I called Dr. Laderas (who thought Ann had my permission to call...) and told her I'd bring Mom in on Monday—or sooner—if she began acting like it was worse than the flu.

Pneumonia is called "the old person's friend." It often comes to a frail person as a secondary infection to a flu, broken hip, a cold, the result of being bedridden after surgery, or another infection. When pneumonia comes, often the person, left untreated, will shortly go into a coma or sleep a lot and die. It's a fairly quick and peaceful exit. I felt this wasn't such a bad way for The Doctor to go. Bronchitis, on the other hand, is not a life-threatening condition, unless it goes into pneumonia. I had thought a lot about where to draw the line in treating her.

Mom is trapped in that body. While I could do nothing to get her out, I'm sure not going to do anything to keep her trapped in there longer than necessary. If she goes into bronchitis we'll treat it; if she gets pneumonia we'll let her go free. I'll check on Mom again tomorrow and Sunday.

This episode was upsetting to me also because I had made a promise to Dad on his deathbed that I intended to keep. Ann knew how I felt. I certainly did not want Mom treated for something she didn't even have just to make sure she wouldn't get it! However, as with any family, disagreements arise, and then it's time to forgive and get on with things.

Mom became the great, great aunt of triplets this winter. Pee Wee's daughter had triplets, and it was fun showing Mom the pictures. She always loved looking at babies. Considering that no fertility drugs were involved, this was a rare and special event for our family, and we celebrated from Texas to Alaska!

By the end of the winter we saw The Doctor begin to lose her ability to walk. One day while out with me, she tripped. Fortunately I had her by the hand, so she didn't fall. Ann said she had also recently tripped in the hallway. Yet two weeks after these incidents, she was again walking like a trooper. Each new behavior, each new problem would start this way. There were sporadic episodes, widely separated. Then they would become more frequent and closer together. Finally, they were constant.

By spring Mom was incontinent of both bowel and bladder. To make matters worse, if she wasn't watched every minute, she would pull down her pants and take off her diaper! She might even "examine" the contents of the diaper. Gross and messy. Ann said she had heard of Alzheimer's patients doing this but always thought it was because they weren't getting good enough care. Now it was happening to one of *her* people. One day she took Mom to the bathroom seven times—and it happened anyway.

Also The Doctor was very busy. She was more agitated than ever. Sometimes she sat in a chair and rocked back and forth. She would no longer nap, something that had been a lifelong habit. Sleep at night became shorter. She often looked tired. We tried increasing her desipramine, but it had a side effect of thickening the saliva and increasing production of it at the higher dosage. I took Mom for a car ride and was grossed out by this saliva junk. Once she tried spitting it out the window with the window closed. I opened the window. I kept giving her napkins and Kleenexes. We came home early.

I called Meredith at the University of Washington to find out what the physicians there were prescribing for agitation. I didn't just want a sedative if there was a better alternative. Meredith gave me the names of two medications, Haldol and Mellaril. I then called Dr. Laderas, described the problems, and gave her the information that Meredith had given me. Thus began a series of trials with medicine to help Mom. Ann tried one. Then another. Then the dosages were modified. Then one was tried with the desipramine. We tried to give Ann some freedom since she was the one who had to deal with The Doctor on a day-to-day basis. I wanted Ann to know that we would do everything we could to help and accommodate her. I wanted Mom to be able to stay with Ann. The problem was that whenever we found something that calmed Mother, it also affected her walk; she staggered, or it made her look and act drugged—or it didn't work at all. Even though Mom was much easier to manage on the medication, Ann did not like the side effects. From the journal:

There are two reasons to prescribe medication. The first is to help the condition of the patient. The second is to help those caring for the patient. Obstetricians, for example, give drugs at one time or another to induce labor. They will do it if a life-threatening condition exists. They do it to help the mother or baby live. Some will also induce labor for their own convenience, so a baby is born before the middle of the night or weekend. Likewise old people are medicated for either their benefit or their caregiver's. Ann is willing to medicate Mother enough so that Mother can rest, so she will sleep at night. She is not willing to medicate her by day to make Mother more easy to care for. I have given Ann permission to medicate Mother mildly by day . . . since she fights Ann and Ana for the morning bathing ritual, etc.

The only good thing that came of all of this experimentation was that I discovered that Health Tek Pharmacy, near and dear to my heart already because of their having a hat to collect urine specimens, also would *deliver* both prescriptions and diapers! After *months* of fiddling around with medicine, we were back to desipramine twice per day with an extra one thrown in if there was reason for it. And the trouble with *that* was that when Mom had enough of it in her to calm her, she would sometimes get the literal gobs of saliva in her mouth that she had to spit up.

6-11-94. I went to see Mom on Wednesday. Ann said the new medicine was not only not working, but might be making the agitation worse! Ann has really been having a hard time with Mom. I think she has wondered if she could continue to keep Mom. She told me she'd like to keep Mom to the end, so we have to find some solutions. I knew this was serious.

There seemed to be no end to these medical issues with heavy ethical overtones to weigh and decide. It would be one thing to do this professionally, but I was in the middle of it with my own family. I found it emotionally wearing. Teaching is also emotionally wearing from time to time, and I felt the effects of carrying a large emotional load all the time.

A boy in my class was suspended this week. It was a rough week all around. However, it was beautiful this afternoon, so Mom and I went for a walk and looked at flowers.

But it was not only problems that came in all shapes and sizes. Solutions did, too. Ann and Ken were able to get away for a short trip to

Reno in late spring. Ann's son, also named Ken, had once run a foster care home, and was licensed, so he filled in for them. After one weekend with The Doctor, he suggested a Geri-Chair, a chair with a tray that snaps in across the front of it—like using a high chair for a baby.

I called my helpful pharmacy and, sure enough, they had a durable equipment division that could help me. I found out that these chairs, technically called table chairs, come in regular and reclining. Ann thought we should get the reclining since The Doctor would eventually be able to use the reclining part if, for example, her circulation got worse. I could either rent or buy the chair, but the rent was high enough for me to decide to buy it. They said they often bought these chairs back used for about half price. Unfortunately they didn't have any used ones available.

Of course I consulted with John and Tom before making a purchase that ran just over $700. Both of them said to buy the chair for Mom. Whatever would help her they would support. Here again, we had to spend money to save money. With The Doctor too agitated even to sit and eat a meal, it was getting more and more difficult for Ann to keep Mom. And the drugs—well they *drugged* Mom. We all decided to go with the chair. I called and had the chair delivered.

In my reading, the experts warned against overuse of restraints, saying they could actually cause *more* agitation. I didn't really think of the Geri-Chair as a restraint, but right from the start we were careful to not overuse it.

But, boy, did it work! Ann used it primarily for Mom's meals. Ann had found that The Doctor did better when eating by herself. She put the Geri-Chair in Mom's room and fed her there. Often left alone, The Doctor could feed herself. Ken said she was able to just focus on her food. Mom gained six pounds in the first couple of months with the chair!

I had a student whose mother was the activity director in an Alzheimer's unit. I asked her what she would suggest for Mom to play with. Mom was so agitated; she needed something to do with her hands. Mrs. Tiller suggested a pat mat (plastic with water and toys inside), Nerf and squish balls, and baby-type toys with beads on a wire to move that won't go anywhere.

I went to K-Mart and found a bead toy and a couple of balls. I couldn't find a pat mat but will keep looking. So many of the baby toys make noise that I don't think she'll like. Also I found some large phonics cards. They are brightly colored and have pictures and letters on them. When I took the things over to her yesterday, we sat for a while and tried some of them, one at a time. Most calming to her were the cards. She could sit with them for hours. She kept trying to force the beads off the plastic wire. She may break that toy. I told Ann that my friend had also said that TV and music can agitate Alzheimer's patients. Ken said sometimes TV calms her, too.

We discovered that dance and music on TV was something The Doctor loved. She also liked old movies—Bing Crosby, Fred Astair, that sort of thing. She liked some Westerns—like re-runs of "The Big Valley." They might have reminded her of growing up on a farm. And she always loved horses. Anything violent or unhappy, tense, or sad was upsetting to her.

Many of my notecards confirmed that The Doctor also still enjoyed outings of all kinds.

1-17-94. I took Mom to the mall with me. It's only a mile from her place, and I needed to get two baby gifts; I knew she'd like being in the baby department. I didn't want to let her ride the escalator down for fear that she'd fall, so we took the stairs, and I held onto her really well. We did take the escalator back up, and I held onto her then, too. Of course she loved the baby department and the little kids with their moms who were also shopping. I was even able to let go of Mom's hand and let her look at all the soft baby things on her own. After a few minutes she was ready to go home, so we did.

2-9-94. Ralph took Mom to the dentist on Tuesday to have her teeth cleaned again. Then, since Janelle was in Vancouver for a horn lesson and had the car, she picked Mom up and took her home while Ralph had his teeth cleaned. Ralph said Mom was really good at the dentist's...Then today I stopped by and brought Mom some shampoo that she needed. She wasn't quite as "far away" as when I saw her last week; when I asked her how she was she said, "Fine!" the first time! When I got up to leave, I got about halfway to the door when I saw Mom get up. I kept going and looked back from outside. She was walking toward the kitchen, having already forgotten why she got up and that I had been there.

3-18-94. We went for a drive today. Although it had rained most of the day, it cleared up for our drive. Spring is here, and there were lots of pretty pink trees to look at. We went out into the country and saw horses, cows, barns and fields—Mom's favorite things still. She sort of "woke up" after a while with me. I sing familiar songs to her and point things out.

3-25-94. I took Mom on a half mile walk around the block. She did very well today. The ornamental plums are in bloom, and she loved all the pink trees. I couldn't believe how well she walked to-day—good pace, too.

4-1-94. As we drove along I sang "She'll Be Comin' 'Round the Mountain When She Comes" to Mom and "Turkey In the Straw" which I "do-do-doed" because I don't know all the words. Mom perks up and looks brighter when I sing some rousing thing.

4-8-94. We went to the craft shop; I needed some ribbon for bows for Heather's wedding. We found some iridescent foil ribbon, and I took that over to the floral and bridal shop. I also tried on a dress there. Mom was very good the whole time. She saw candy bars at the craft shop and sort of hung around them, so I bought her a Milky Way. Then there was a bowl of peppermints at the bridal shop, and she helped herself! It's been kind of a stormy day, so we didn't walk outdoors much.

4-14-94. I stopped by as usual after work and Mom was in a ready-

to-go mood. It was a gorgeous afternoon, so we went for a half-mile walk around the block and then did it again halfway! She was really walking well today and came out with several coherent phrases and even a couple of sentences! Once she said something that was a total jumble and started to laugh. I laughed too and said, "That didn't quite come out right, did it?" Today she knew it for a moment and it struck her as funny. So many things are in bloom now. The tulips in her neighborhood are especially bright so we looked closely at some and ooo-ed and aaah-ed.

4-29-94. I took her shopping with me. I needed to get her Mother's Day gift and a baby gift and a couple of plants. She loves flowers and babies, so I knew she'd like this outing. In the Baby Department, sure enough, was a baby. I said to the young couple, "Do you mind if she says hello to your baby? She has Alzheimer's, but she still loves babies." Of course young parents love to have someone else appreciate their baby, so Mom got to smile at him and touch him, and when he smiled back at her, she really lit up and said, "Where is your mama? Where is your daddy?"—just as clear as a bell. They couldn't even tell she had Alzheimer's for a moment! Then we went on and we managed to find a sack of chocolate covered mints that she didn't want to part with so we got that, too. I got her nylons for the wedding, and we got a few flowers. After that we drove around a little, so she could see some gardens.

5-6-94. I took Mom for a drive. We had to go to the Health Tek Pharmacy to pick up more diapers. The inserts don't work well. [Even though Ann was getting up twice each night to change Mom, her diapers were soaking through at night. Overnight diapers for adults were not available, so we tried a couple of different inserts that were made to help this.]

Then we went to Fred Meyer's to buy some fuchsias and bedding plants. Mom tried to take her pants down while we were looking (I think she had to go to the bathroom), and she also kept taking the little plastic markers out of the plants to put in her pants. I have to hold one of her hands and move the cart with the other. She loves flowers but missed the point today. She took a package of gum off a shelf when we were checking out and opened it. So I bought it and gave her a piece and hoped we wouldn't end up with gum all over everything. On the way back I sang to her and held her hand to tap the beat, and for a moment she did it herself today—the first time in months that she has been able to do that.

7-12-94. I took Mom for a long walk today, and then we went for a drive in the country. It was a beautiful day to sing "Summertime" and "Zip-A-Dee-Doo-Dah." Mom smiles when I sing though she can no longer sing with me or keep a beat.

9-15-94. The Doctor was having another good day. We went to Kunze Farms, our usual place, where she shoplifted with abandon, and I told the lady there that I'd pay for what she picked up. She selected a couple of apples. I bought those plus a sackful to take back to Ann. We also got some tomatoes, plums, and hazel nut brittle, a candy both Ann and Mom like. Then we went driving around while she ate her apples and some candy. Back at Ann's I gave her the loot, and she had some peaches, so she swapped those with me.

We're having beautiful fall weather. Ann said that Mom has wanted to be outdoors a lot. She has spent quite a bit of time in the yard the last couple of days.

10-21-94. Took Mom for a lovely fall evening drive. She was pretty far gone tonight until I suggested that we find a couple of "fellas" and go out dancing! That really brightened her up! She even did a little two-step when I returned her to Ann and told Ann about it!

These are just samples of The Doctor's outings. Ann saw to it that she walked regularly, weather permitting. I took her out also each and every week at least.

By the beginning of 1994, The Doctor Agnes, K.E., had begun to babble not in words, but in nonsense syllables, much as a baby does. She would often repeat the same syllable again and again. By the end of the year, actual words were seldom coming from her. Sentences were rare:

I was sitting next to Mom on the sofa talking to Ann. The TV was on and Mom was babbling as usual. Suddenly Mom nudged me and said with a laugh, "You're not even listening to me!" I laughed and said, "You're right!" Just as suddenly, she was "gone" again.

Sometimes I could get her to speak a little Norwegian. I might count to ten in Norwegian, and she would start in. Even the nonsense syllables sometimes had a Norwegian accent. Often she would say, "Nay, nay, nay" and sound very Scandinavian.

The Doctor was frequently in her own world as she babbled, unaware of others in the room. She would come out of it when directly spoken to:

Mom was lying down when I came. Ann and I went into her room. Mom's eyes were closed, but they opened and she started quietly mumbling. Ann and I stood by her bed for a few minutes talking. Mom showed no response to us until Ann bent over her and called her name, "Agnes, Agnes, your daughter is here." Then Mom sort of woke up from her stupor, and we helped her up.

Sometimes when I talked to her, she talked back with the wrong words but the right expression and the right tone to her voice—like she was really conversing, even understanding, but the words were wrong, that's all. Some days it was not even that much. She mumbled along, but it wasn't in *response* to what I said. She was having her own conversations.

Once on a walk she said, "Are you cold?" I said, "No, are you?" She only mumbled something, but I knew that she was and took her home. On another walk she was mumbling along and out popped, "Puss, puss." I looked around and, sure enough, there was a cat! Mom never got past being a back-seat driver, either. She would still manage to say at intersections, "Be careful!" Ann said she did this even when she took Mom out.

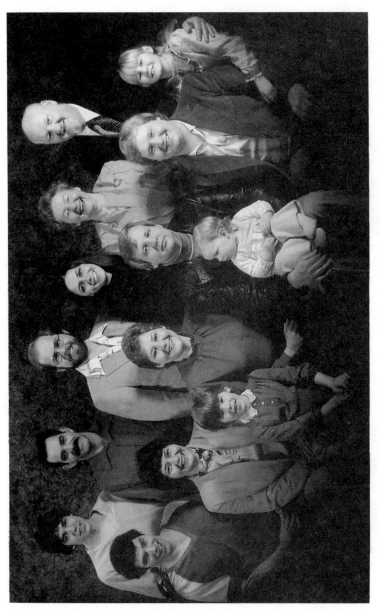

The Leonard Family in 1982 (L-R). Top: Eric Stowell, Arne Stowell, Ralph Akin, Denise Leonard, Agnes Leonard, Chuck Leonard. Bottom: John Stowell, Mary Lou Stowell, Janelle Akin, Charlotte Akin, John & Natalie Leonard, Tom Leonard, Heather Akin.

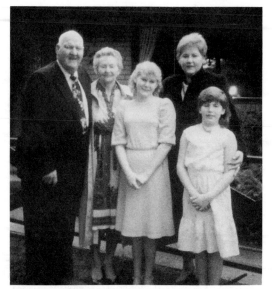

Easter 1986 with the author and grand-
daughters, Heather and Janelle, in Spokane
(Early Confusional Stage).

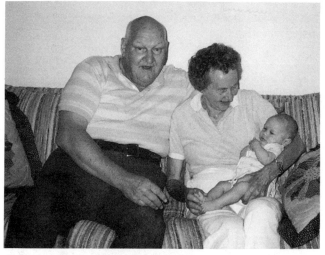

In Kansas with grandnephew, 1987.

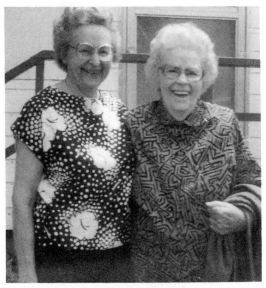

Agnes Leonard and sister, Dagny, in Idaho, 1988 (Early Confusional Stage).

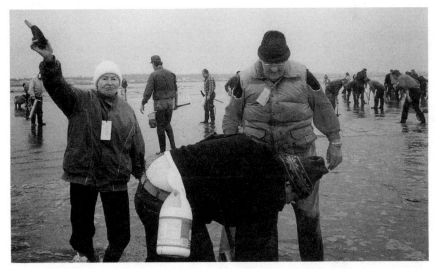

Clam digging at the ocean, spring 1990 (Middle Dementia Stage).

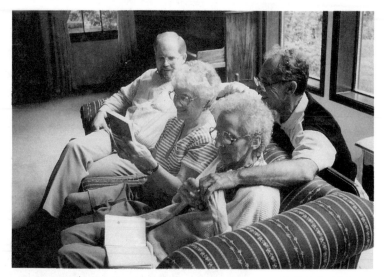

Agnes's 78th birthday at the home of the author, with Ralph Akin
and Betty and Homer Schmitt, 1994 (Late Dementia Stage).

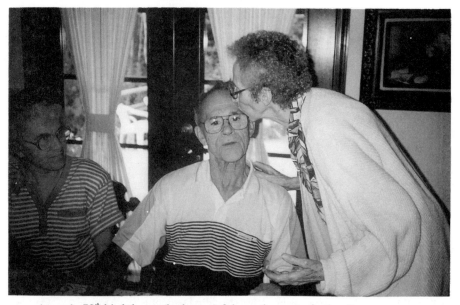

Agnes's 78th birthday at the home of the author, comforting "poor
Homer" with a kiss (Late Dementia Stage).

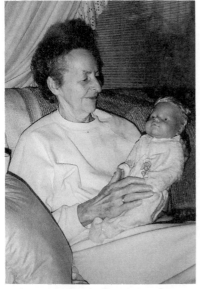

Agnes at Ann's foster care home with baby doll. Note the "Afro" perm (Late Dementia Stage).

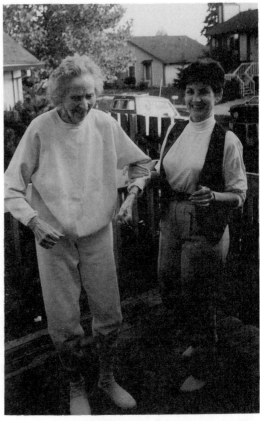

Dancing with Ann on the deck of her foster care home (Late Dementia Stage).

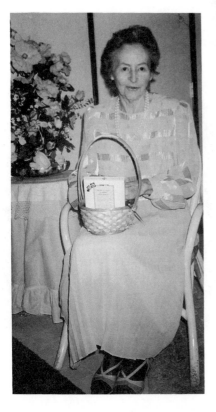

In foster care at Ann's house, Easter 1993. Note child-like demeanor (Late Dementia Stage).

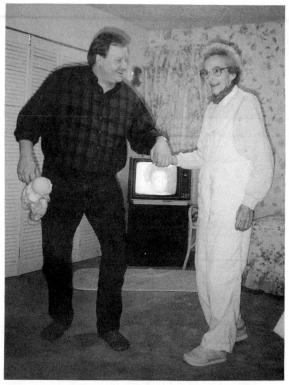

Dancing with Tom, January 1995.
Note custom pink overalls. Tom
holds baby (Late Dementia Stage).

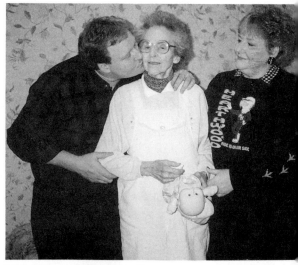

With Tom and Charlotte, January
1995 (Late Dementia Stage).

Mom also communicated in ways other than words. When Ann discovered that The Doctor ate better on her own, she explained to me that when Mom was with people she was always getting up, wanting to "fuss and do." Ann concluded, "I bet she was a wonderful hostess, wasn't she?"

And she was! Dad always wanted people around—he was your basic party animal. Mom got tired of being a hostess all the time—but she was good at it!

Here was The Doctor, slow of walk, incontinent, babbling like a baby yet still able to communicate something very essential about her personality—she was a wonderful hostess; she liked people; she was accommodating. Every day of her life she was *proving* it! *She was still in there.*

Once The Doctor, Ann, and I were sitting on the couch. She pretended suddenly like she was asleep and Ann said, "Yes, I know you're tired now." I left shortly after that.

She also gave every indication of being able to understand more than she could say. Ralph and I were out running errands one day and took Mom along. When we got to the paint store, she had been in the front seat, and I was in the back. Ralph said as I got out, "Are you sure you want to take her in?" I didn't see Mom's reaction. But Ralph said she had been hurt by his remark—it had deflated her. He thought she seemed sad after that. Fortunately I had said matter of factly, "Oh, she'll be fine" as I had gotten out of the car. And she was OK.

The Doctor Agnes, K.E., never tired of a joke. One day after running another errand, she and I were on the way home: She was babbling along, and she put up three fingers and said, "Three!" Then she put one finger down, then another finger down, and then she got a funny look on her face. I said, "You're not giving me the finger are you?!" And she laughed and knew the joke. I said, "Here I come and take you out for a nice ride and you give me the finger?!" She laughed and knew she'd been naughty.

In spite of her misbehavior on a variety of levels, I did talk to her about Heaven when we went for rides. I knew she could still understand some and I wanted her to know she had my permission to die. So one day I was telling her this. I told her I was proud of her. I knew she worked deliberately at being cheerful still. I told her she had fought the good fight. I complimented her for her courage with this disease that can rob the mind but never the dignity of one who fights on through the mists to be loving to others. I was quiet, thinking: *Her time has come. I can't bear watching her deteriorate much longer.* Then she said, "Well, Charlotte, we've had some good times, haven't we?" It's always a shock when something so coherent comes out. But I said, "Yes, we have."

She hadn't called me by name in years and never would again.

One of the unfolding miracles of taking care of The Doctor was finding and being able to admit that there was joy in this task.

It is OK for me to enjoy taking care of Mother. It is OK to admit that she can still be fun and funny and that I can love and enjoy her. When I tell her we'll go out dancing and she wiggles her hips—she is so cute and funny even now. She is so affectionate and kissy. She always wants a kiss. I love taking her on walks and rides, much the same as I enjoyed this when Heather and Janelle were young.

There is more to this than just playing the tired, dutiful, stressed martyr role. There is, also, the joy of it.

Some days I think it is time for her to go; I am ready. Her life has no more purpose or meaning. Then I learn something about transcending from her like I did today—and it makes me know how short-sighted and foolish I am—how glad I am that her life is not in my hands or hers, but God's.

Life was in full swing for the Leonard and Akin families. John sold the house in January. It was a big load off him. He no longer had to make periodic trips to Seattle to take care of it. The house was alternately a financial and emotional drain. We were all both happy and sad that it had sold. John invested the proceeds in mutual funds with a regular payment plan to Ann for The Doctor's care.

From a February 1994 entry:

I'm swamped right now at school and at home. Janelle did well at her audition last weekend.

The sale of Mom's house in Seattle went through this week.

Heavy sigh. John plans to give an updated accounting to us.
Although we could now settle Dad's half of the estate, we're going
to leave it together until Mom goes. It is the right thing to do all
around—ensures good care for her. She can primarily live off the
interest and Social Security. By doing that, the value of her half of
the estate does not erode—leaving us with potentially more in the
long run.

Taking The Doctor to the dentist for her quarterly cleaning was becoming a mega-event. Once in the dentist's chair, she got so tired of fighting the hygienist, that she simply turned over on her side, right in the chair, and kind of curled up into a fetal position. The hygienist kept on working. Mom was sweet, but she didn't want to be messed with.

Ralph did a better job with Mom at the dentist. Partly because she always liked men, we think. It may be that he calmed her more. Even when I took her, she settled down and brightened when Dick came in to check on her.

The Doctor Agnes, K.E., also bruised easily. It didn't help her to fight when people needed to bathe her or help her go to the bathroom. She didn't understand that and so had an occasional bruise. Having tried to dress her a time or two myself, I understood that this was somewhat unavoidable. If we were careful with her, it wasn't bad at all, and it was certainly better than having her drugged.

As spring came, my family was facing all kinds of milestones. Janelle graduated from high school, Ralph and I celebrated our twenty-fifth wedding anniversary, and preparations for a wedding were under way:

5-21-94. I didn't stay long. We're in the middle of Janelle's
graduation plans and Heather's wedding next month. In addition,
the close of the school year is always so busy for me.

I generally see Mom once a week any more, sometimes twice
if she's not feeling well or needs something. On top of that, I run
her errands, correspond with her friends, call and update her
family and closest friends, balance her checkbook, and buy her
gifts (for grandchildren, etc.) It all takes time. It's a lifesaver for

me to have her so well cared for that I don't really need to be there all the time.

Tom and Teri were planning on coming from Anchorage for Heather's wedding, and Tom wanted to see The Doctor. Teri suggested that I send pictures of Mom—several so that they could get a good look at her and not be shocked when they came.

5-28-94. Tom and Teri were shocked at her pictures. She looks so frail. I told Tom to get used to them because she does look like that. I want him to be able to greet her with a big hug and a smile. Heather, Ann, and I decided that we're going to have Mom skip the wedding and just come to the reception.

6-2-94. I'm totally swamped right now at school. I told a teacher friend today I had no idea how I was going to get report cards done in 1 week! Heather's wedding is in three weeks. Janelle's high school graduation is this next week. And we have a wedding in Olympia to go to this weekend. Gasp. I hope nothing flares up with Mom!

6-11-94. We also celebrated our 25th anniversary this week. Last night Janelle graduated from high school. Ralph helped chaperone the all-night party. The wedding is in two weeks. Every time I turn around, there are more details. School will be out next Tuesday, and so everything is a zoo there, too. When it rains, it pours.

6-15-94. With all the milestones going on around here, money matters concern me. When Heather graduated from high school, Dad gave her $750.00 for part of her trip to Europe. So do I give Janelle $750? Or do I give her nothing? Dad gave Janelle money at the same time as Heather's graduation. She used it to help buy her French horn. The reason Dad gave such generous gifts was that he'd given John and Tom some money or forgiven some loan or something. He wanted to give me money, but I wouldn't take it.

Ralph and I decided early in our marriage not to get involved with friends or family in financial matters. I said, "If you want to give your money away, give it to your grandchildren." So—what to do for Janelle's graduation now? She is, after all, the only grandchild who has actually suffered because of the time I've had to put into Mom. I decided to compromise and gave her $200.00 [from Mom's account] *which I had John approve.*

Then when Heather and I were going over wedding details, she mentioned that both of Marc's grandmothers had given them $100.00. So do I give Heather and Marc money from Mom? I've been very careful not to take financial advantage of Mother. I shouldn't pad my children's pockets at her expense. Anyway, I've decided to give Heather and Marc $100.00. Then for birthdays this year I'm going to give the other younger grandchildren each $100.00 from Mom's account. I'll get permission from John and Tom over all of this.

I'm still agonizing over what to do with Mother at the wedding. I talked to Mom's sister, Babe, last weekend by phone. My philosophy has always been that this is part of life, like infancy, pregnancy, etc. You don't cloister these people. They need and enjoy the moment, being out among others. Babe had a totally different slant on it. She said having Mom at even the reception would ruin the memory and the wedding for John and Tom and probably their children, not to mention other friends. She also said that Mom did not need to be the object of pity, that (brainless) she shouldn't be paraded around other people, that she would never have wanted that for herself back when she had her mind. To do so now would ruin memories of her; it would be demeaning and an injustice to her. I asked John, Ann, and Ralph about this, and they all agreed with at least part of it! Then I asked Heather, the bride. She said she'd be fine with Mom not coming. She was a little worried about it. I said, "Well, that settles it. I had thought you wanted her there." She said, "Well, I knew you did." Therefore, Mom is not coming to the wedding or reception but Ken and Ann will come.

I still struggled with this. Of course I took The Doctor out and about. She enjoyed it and generally she was either with family or with total strangers, like when we went into grocery stores or whatever. We weren't among people who had known her, either friends, acquaintances, or family. That seemed OK to me. In wanting her to be at the wedding, I was thinking of how thrilled she would be at the sight of it—even though she would not remember it.

> *6-20-94 I talked to Homer and Betty today to get more wedding advice regarding Mom. It still isn't settled within me. They both agreed she should not go at all after I presented all sides. Homer said the reason was that if it could make one guest uncomfortable (John especially and his family) then she shouldn't be there. Betty said if it were her, and she could choose now with her mind, she wouldn't want others to see her like that. So now I think it really is settled. At least for today.*
>
> *Heather and Marc fly in tonight. The music rehearsal is today. The wedding is only five days away. Things are going to start popping around here!*

The wedding was on June 25th.

> *6-26-94. To paraphrase Isadora Duncan: "If I could tell you what I am thinking, there would be no reason to dance."*
>
> *I ran across that when the girls were small. Janelle was taking dance lessons. I even included it in a collage I made of the girls. Then I forgot about it until today.*
>
> *The wedding was yesterday. Ken and Ann came, but we left Mom home. I'll always feel bad about that decision. The only other way was no better. It was a beautiful, small country wedding—just as Heather wanted. Heather never looked more beautiful. Janelle's music came together. The horse and carriage ride from the church to our home was the frosting on the cake.*
>
> *I didn't sleep much last night. Ann called this morning to say that Mom was having a good day, so I took Tom and Teri over to*

see her. She did a double take when she saw Tom. They were always so close. He gave her a big hug and a kiss. She kissed him time and again. And then she began to dance! Just a few short steps, but her joy was unmistakable. We took her for a short walk. As we headed down the ramp in front of Ann's, she danced again. Tom said to me, "Is this usual?!" He was laughing. I said, "Well, she's happy to see you!" ("If I could tell you what I am thinking, there would be no reason to dance...") On the walk she held our hands and she would bring his hand up and kiss it every now and then. Tom wanted his daughter, Jessie, to see her granny, so we took her with us when we left. She sat in front with Tom and gave him her hand for a kiss every now and then. She never called him by name or said much coherent, but it was clear that she loved him and knew he was a big part of her life. It really tickled Tom. He could also see what a wonderful home she lives in. He watched her go on the back deck and putter. He wondered if she could go out there by herself and Ann assured him she could. She has some freedom within structure. The deck has a gate and is locked. Tom saw her room and a couple of other residents. It was a good time....Tom and Teri took Mom to see Jessie back at my house then. Jessie didn't really know how to relate to Granny. It was OK—not terrible. They took Mom back home after five to ten minutes. Teri and Tom were glad they saw her. I was relieved.

Babe wishes she had not seen Mom. I think John feels the same way. It's impossible for me to know how someone else will relate and respond to seeing Mom. So it is impossible to tell someone whether they should come and see her. I get asked all the time by friends and relatives alike. Tom said he'd like to see her each time he comes down from Anchorage.

Tom had even liked how Mom was dressed—in a cute sweatshirt and matching sweat pants. She had several outfits like that. In addition, Ann kept her so beautiful, trimming her nails, fixing her hair, lotioning her hands. She always looked good.

After the wedding was over and all the guests left, it was time to do two things with the rest of the summer. We had to get Janelle ready for school in New York in the fall. She had been accepted at the University of Rochester. It was also time to start writing about The Doctor.

And it was time for another birthday.

8-7-94. Mom's 78th birthday. We had Homer and Betty here with Mom for a champagne luncheon. Ann and Ken were invited too, but couldn't get away. Ana's husband likes Ana with their family on Sundays. He works all week, and Ana works on Saturdays so Ann can go shopping with Ken. It's understandable. Ann's son, Ken, also was not available. Janelle picked Mom up after church and brought her back to our house for the luncheon.

Mom wasn't having a great day. Not a glimmer of real recognition of Homer and Betty. She did kiss them though, and she told Betty she loved her. Mom's walk was unsteady and slow. She wet her pants some, and I finally understood that she had to go to the bathroom, so I took her in and set her on the toilet so she could go. Ann had sent a couple of diapers, so I put a new one on her—first time I had done that! (It was easy to do this right when Mom was on the toilet—not a big deal at all.)

She ate only part of her meal. She kept wanting to get up and fidget. I can understand why her Geri-Chair helps her eat. We gave her lemonade instead of champagne. I wasn't sure what alcohol would do with her medication. The festivity of the occasion also was over Mom's head.

Janelle didn't stay for lunch, so it was just Ralph and I, Homer and Betty, and Mom.

Betty said for the first time that seeing Mom made her feel like crying. It has been hard for her to watch; she has been such a true and faithful friend.

As we talked after lunch, Homer said he was sure Mom was still able to understand even though you couldn't tell by looking at her or by her speech. We talked about this a while, and then he looked over at Mom and said in a wailing, sad, poor-me tone, "I don't think anybody loves me at all! Nobody loves me!" Mom went right over to him and gave him a kiss! He did it a while later, and she did the same thing.

We had a little walk to the creek—slowly, slowly—before we had cake and ice cream—which Mom did eat!

Then Homer and Betty left, and I took Mom back home and put her to bed for a nap.

There won't be a 79th birthday party. If Mom lives that long, she won't be able to make the trip here, probably won't be able to walk. It had been five months since H and B had seen Mom—longer than ever before! They could see quite a decline in her since the beginning of March.

I was only partly right.

The Doctor Agnes, K.E., continued to be part of the Alzheimer's research at the University of Washington. Each month I sent in a report. Their funding had been cut, so they weren't able to send someone to continue the testing of Mom. I called and asked if I could pay for the testing and have one of their psychometrists come privately, on their own time. I would be happy to share results. They agreed.

One day in August, Zilpha Haycox came to test The Doctor. I listened around the corner (see Appendix B for Zilpha's report and test results).

8-12-94. I had a wonderful lunch with Zilpha! We solved all the world's problems. "The best nursing home care is not nearly as good as good foster care," she told me. She cried at the thought of those she sees in nursing homes.

Zilpha was the University of Washington's lead psychometrist. She had a case load of hundreds. She was a pro who had seen care in all forms. She felt deeply and emotionally about the majority of "care" she saw regarding Alzheimer's. Zilpha's job took her into the daily lives of people, into their homes or into their nursing homes. It is a different perspective than what a doctor would have who has patients come to him or her. Zilpha saw the environment that the patient came from.

8-13-94. One of the other things Zilpha mentioned was that it is wrong for caregivers to talk in front of Alzheimer's patients about them—just because the Alzheimer's patients do understand much more that we ever give them credit for.

As I went back to visit Mom after I had lunch with Zilpha, I caught myself and Ann doing just that.

Zilpha also said that Mom was infantile, the way she held out her arms to greet people. She also noted that Mom's face is losing expression, although she still does smile.

Zilpha asked about Mom and our family during lunch. She had suspected that Mom was very sociable; those who are sociable hide Alzheimer's the best and longest. Zilpha said she'll test people who say just the right things when she meets them, who are warm and outgoing. When they take the test, she finds huge gaps in what they know and can do.

We talked about the importance of the research, Zilpha saying that when there is a strong genetic link, it ruins the lives of the people in those families as they must live just waiting their turn. Sadly, this is most often the case when the age of onset is so young—between 45 and 55.

Mom scored two on the test. She was having a really good day, and Zilpha even said she could easily have scored zero. The Doctor got a point when Zilpha handed her a paper telling her to take it with her right hand. Mom, being right handed, did. Then, since Mom is folding everything right now, she got another point because Zilpha told her to fold it! She could do nothing else, even on simpler tests.

The journey back in time continued for The Doctor. Her dancing became more like the bounce-dancing a very young child does to music. A child that has just learned to walk will kind of bounce in rhythm with body and knees when music is played. The Doctor also held her hands up and out when I came in the room. It had the look of a one-year-old holding out arms to be picked up. I could even put her on my lap if I was sitting in the dining room talking to Ann. She would just sit there as we visited.

Otherwise she would get into everything. My notes documented the changes that happened throughout the year.

Ann said that one day last week Mom told her she was a little girl. Most of Mom's gestures are now infantile, especially the way she holds up her arms to greet Ann. It is the same gesture a baby gives its mother to be picked up.

Another entry:

Throws her food like a baby in a high chair. Throws glass down. Threw a blouse at Nina.

While she might be calmed by the voice of a man, she no longer flirted, not even in the way a little three-year-old girl flirts.

12-17-94. Homer—however hard he tried—couldn't get Mom to be sweet to him. She made faces at him and said, "No" if he asked her if she loved him and so forth. He was really cute with her, but she was a deliberate stinker. She was sharper today, though, than she was in August when they last saw her. I still think she is losing the ability to smile. When they got up to leave, Homer went to hug Mom, and she kind of poked him in the tummy—an obvious tease from her.

The demeanor of The Doctor was like that of a one- to two-year-old or younger during this period. The incontinence and unsteady walk added to this effect. The speech that was often in babble, but sometimes in words or short sentences, did too. Even the way The Doctor was kissy and affectionate was now like that of a very young child.

Likewise, the care Mother needed resembled the care needed for an infant or toddler. She needed help being fed, dressed, and bathed. She needed to be watched and needed toys to play with. She needed a loving home with one-on-one care, someone paying attention to her because she couldn't verbally express a need.

The Doctor remained the most permanent resident at Annabelle's Foster Care. After Christine was hospitalized for pneumonia Mr. Philips arrived. He also had a stroke; both his speech and walk were impaired.

> *He is a gentleman and told me how sweet Mom is when I met him.*
> *Mom goes over to him and gives him a pat or a kiss periodically.*
> *Ken got a new surround speaker system that he was setting up.*
> *He's a great guy, too. I've grown so fond of Ann and Ken.*

Besides being a former history teacher, Ken was an electrician profession-ally and a handyman for Ann's business. He once re-wired the master bathroom light switch in the house because Nina would go in there at night, turn off the light when she was done—and be "lost." Ken wired it so that the light was permanently on. Ken had also converted a double garage into an apartment for himself and Ann. He later converted that to two rooms. He also did yard work, re-doing most of the back yard when he and Ann bought a large fifth wheeler that also could double as an apartment for people who helped. Ken was seldom without a project.

Ann gave my name out occasionally when someone asked for a reference. Of course I gave rave reviews of the care The Doctor was getting. In January I got a call from someone looking for a place for a 98-year-old friend. Pearl, whom we called Grandma, even though she wasn't a grandmother, soon moved in. Sharp as a tack, she could care for herself. Pearl had recently had cataract surgery. She was just old enough to need someone else to cook and clean for her. Sometimes Ann had people recovering from surgery or a stroke. They would just stay a short time until they could go home and either care for themselves or be more easily cared for by their also-aging spouse. Mr. Philips stayed only a short time. Ann's rates varied depending on the level of care. Someone like Pearl was much easier to care for than The Doctor, so Ann charged accordingly. (Ann raised her price for The Doctor again by $200 in 1994.) Pearl told me the first time I met her that Ann and Ken were "good people—the best." I was always happy to see people move in who felt lucky to be there, who appreciated their new home. Pearl was one of those.

Often, like a college dorm, the ladies shared clothing:

The ladies at Ann's share clothes. Sometimes people leave clothes with Ann when someone has passed away. A few weeks ago I noticed Mom with different shoes on. I asked Ann about it, and she said they were Nina's. Then last week I noticed that Nina had on Mom's pink and white Cannon Beach sweat shirt. I said to Ann, "I guess it's share and share alike around here!" She said she tried to keep Nina out of Mom's clothes but couldn't always. I told her that if Nina got a little pleasure out of wearing something of Mom's, it was OK with me. Mom wears a good-looking green jacket that someone left behind. It's heavier than the new ones I bought for her, and she needs that now. Ann's generosity letting her wear it saves me going out and buying another (which is time and money), so I guess we can share, too. Ann takes beautiful care of the clothes. They are always clean and in perfect repair. All the people at Ann's look well-kept in clean clothes with their hair combed, and so on. She doesn't always have them "dolled up"—usually it's just neat, clean, and comfy, like her home. The licensing lady came by this past week and told Ann that she had such a happy home. Many are not like that, she said, with people angry or shouting and so on.

Ann said that her home has its moments, too. One day last week Nina was rubbing her leg as if it hurt. Ann said to her, "Did you hurt your leg?" Nina said, "Go to hell! I'm leaving!" With that, Nina got up and walked out the front door. Since Ann was talking with Edna's family [Edna was a new resident], *she sent Ana after Nina.*

Ana was a small woman, middle-aged, and a steady worker. When not working at Annabelle's Foster Care, she was working on things at her own home across the street. She had four children, ranging in age from kindergartners through high schoolers. Ana was a rock-solid person, totally dependable, firm, and kind. She was not given to fuss and frills. I'm sure when Ann sent her after Nina, that Ana was doing her very best.

Ana apparently would try to take Nina's arm and steer her back home at which point Nina would hit Ana! A neighbor saw this and called the police. The police brought Nina and Ana back, where Nina told the police not to drink the coffee because it was drugged! She went on about poisoned food and beatings, and Ann said it was all she could do not to laugh out loud, but she knew at the time it would only enrage Nina. I said, "The police didn't believe any of this I hope?!" Ann said no, she thought they were still having a laugh over it at the station house though. Since then, Nina is back to her usual self with hardly a cross word!

I think the key to discerning a good home is taking in the whole picture. I wouldn't want to do anything but trust what Mom tells me; I've made a point of believing her. However, if the story was usually one way, that's the way I'll believe her. When she began to lose weight I was concerned. Someone said to me, "What does everyone else who lives there look like? What does the lady who has been there a while look like? What do the owners look like? Taste the food." It was good advice, and I knew right away that the problem lay elsewhere. Nevertheless, when it was first happening I made a point of taking Mom home with me for a day at a time a few times—where I cooked her favorite foods. She barely touched her food and wouldn't eat when I fed her.

Ann had two more ladies arrive in the spring. One of the ladies didn't pay much—Medicaid. Ann said she normally wouldn't take her, but the woman was inseparable from her friend, so they moved in together.

That brought the total to five: The Doctor, Nina, Pearl, and the two new ladies. Ann never had more than five at a time. She had more extra help with that many, too.

There was never any question who was the stinker in the bunch though.

Ann said that Mom went to her room one day, lifted the mattress off and sat down and peed on the box springs! Ana had since shampooed it. I told Ann if Mom ever really wrecked anything, I'd replace it.

Mom was not the only problem, however:

Of Ann's five ladies, one is a "troublemaker." They sit down to dinner, and thirty minutes later this one gets them all believing that they haven't eaten yet! Have I said before that Ann and Ken are saints?!

The "troublemaker" was one of the two who came together. She didn't stay long. After she fell a couple of times, her doctor told the family she did not have long to live, so they decided to take her home for the end. Ann said both days and nights were easier without her; she kept everyone stirred up. Her walker woke everyone up at night when she went to the bathroom, and by day she'd have all the ladies wanting to leave! She would get them wanting to go shopping or out to lunch! Her friend, Edna, stayed though.

The Doctor was difficult to manage because her brain was dying. Still, she really fought to be "a good girl." Even though she did things that were difficult to manage, all of Ann's help honored her because she was never purposefully ornery. It was clear, somehow, that she was innocent and brave. She was actually respected still for who she was. Careful and neat in so many ways, it was obvious that accidents with food and bathroom problems were not really about her; they were about the disease. Agitation and spells of crying likewise were easily viewed as part of the disease. The part that was The Doctor fought to be cheerful and fun and sweet. Somehow everyone knew and understood this. Pearl was impatient and had a hard time putting up with Mom's busyness. She would growl at Mom occasionally. Even so, there was an innate dignity to The Doctor that was clearly perceived by all. The Doctor was the lovey in the bunch. It was she who could be counted on for a kiss or a pat whenever she passed by. Even Pearl still liked to be patted and loved. So The Doctor, because she loved others, was loved in return.

It was also important to accommodate Ann and Ken. Ann was careful about who stayed in their home. People who wouldn't make an effort to work with her didn't last long. Edna was becoming more agitated and occasionally violent. By mid year:

Edna wanders a lot and is violent sometimes. Ann asked Edna's family if she could put her in the Geri-Chair now and then. They said, "No way!" Ann suggested that they take Edna home for a day to see the need. Like a mother with a house full of small children, Ann needs to be able to go to the bathroom or run out and get the mail and have her people safe. Edna's family refused to try it for a day saying, "That's what we're paying you for!" Ann has given them thirty days to move Edna. These people will pay twice as much to put Edna in the only nursing home in the area with a bed available right now. Not the best around, it has been in the papers for violations repeatedly in the past six months. Their foolishness appalls me. What if it were they? Wouldn't they want an accommodation or two made, so they could stay in Ann's comfortable home? The nursing home will sedate and confine Edna and that will be the end of it!

I go out of my way to treat Ann well. I got her a gardenia corsage for her birthday to wear when she and Ken went out for dinner. [I had given them a gift certificate for dinner out for Mother's Day. Ann's birthday was just a couple of weeks later.] *Actually it was paid for from Mom's account. When Ann tells me she needs something for Mom, I get it right away. Partly this is because I know Ann well enough by now to trust her. At first I didn't, though, and I would bring Mom home with me for a day at a time. Just to check.*

It made me both mad and sad to see people have to leave because families were unwilling to work with Ann to help their loved one. Sometimes it was a need to change medication and work with the doctor. Sometimes it was a case of damage to Ann's home. Whatever Mom needed, whatever Ann felt was best, I wanted to make sure we were working together, so The Doctor could stay in the comfortable home where she was tended and loved. In reference to trying medication changes to help sleep and decrease agitation:

6-30-94. Ken and Ann went canoeing and camping for the weekend. The younger Ken is in charge and Ana helps him. He said Mom's doing well, not agitated today, and she slept all night last night. Finally! *This has taken six weeks or so.* Whew! *I'm lucky Ann has been so patient. Sleep disorders are the number one reason Alzheimer's patients land in nursing homes. Ann knows that I'll do what I can to help her.*

There were many charming things about the home that I came to love. Ann would sometimes have her "beauty shop" going in the summer with all the ladies on the deck, fixing their hair. In the winter Ken often had a big fire in the living room fireplace. Both silk and real flowers forever decorated the dining room table. It was the small things that made this a home.

7-6-94. "Grandma" Pearl and Nina were napping when Mom and I got back from our walk. Ann says that this is her time of day with Mom. She and Mom putter in the yard or kitchen then. I remarked that it was like having a house full of children and you schedule each one some special time. She agreed.

7-18-94. I took Mom for a walk today. Another beautiful day, but she got so hot and tired I was afraid we wouldn't make it back to the house! When we got back Ann had a salad lunch ready for her—tossed green salad with ranch dressing and a Jell-O and cottage cheese salad. Mom ate well while Ann and I visited.

Ann got a new carpet—a beautiful turquoise. She is putting vinyl in Mom's and Nina's room though. Easier to keep clean.

7-22-94. I stopped by in the morning and took Mom for a walk. She had a new plaid short-sleeved shirt on. (We have been having 100-degree weather.) Nina also had a new yellow outfit on. Ann said that she had been to Value Village and found these things for a dollar a piece. The blouse Mom had on matched her green pants perfectly!

Ann and Ken took a trip to Mexico in the fall. Hazel, Ann's sister from Oklahoma, came again to help. I enjoyed getting to know Hazel; she was what I'd call a "good old girl." She reminded me of my Auntie Ethel. Just a salt-of-the-earth type.

Ann and Ken made a big decision in the fall. They bought another home, one for them to live in. I had many mixed feelings, but could surely understand their need for rest. They had grandchildren but were working night and day. Of course they were keeping the business and Ann would still be there during the days—most of Mom's awake time. It was still a change to adjust to.

11-18-94. Ann has hired another new person, so Ann will only be there three day-shifts per week. I'm not wild about all these shifts of people. No one is individually responsible for Mom's care with six or seven people caring for her. So far there's Ann, Ana, Ana's Romanian friend, Sunshine, and the new lady. I guess that's five.

I just finished a night class this week, so I'll have more time to make drop-in visits. I'm going to try to visit four or five times in the next week. I'm also going to weigh Mom this next week.

12-2-94. I had a chance to visit with Ann. Her help, new routine, and new home are all settling into place. She, Ana, and Georgiana (Ana's Romanian friend) each take shifts, and so each has time off, too. It seems to be working out.

That was what finally came to be the routine—about three people working there. Five never really worked out. Ann and Ana and the third changed a few times before getting more settled in 1995.

Another change came in late fall when Nina got the flu. She had Parkinson's in addition to Alzheimer's. Her decline was much more rapid than The Doctor's, as a result. She had a rough time recovering from the flu, being bedridden for a while and then nearly so for a while longer. Her mind was sharper still than The Doctor's. I hated to see Nina so sick, having come to love her.

As December rolled around, I wrote again to Mom's family and friends:

Dear Friends,

Mom continues to live in the foster care home she has been in now for nearly three years. She is so loved and tended there. She is very childlike and content, holding out her arms to welcome visitors.

Mom has very little verbal ability. She is mostly incoherent. She understands more than she can say. Still, she manages to get her point across. When Tom came to visit her from Alaska last June, she took one look at him and began to dance! As we left the house, taking her for a walk, she stopped again, looked at him, and began to dance. He started to giggle and said, "Is this usual?" I said, "No. She's just so happy to see you."

Mom continues to be remarkably healthy. She got a touch of the flu last winter for the first time in over three years. She was fully recovered in about five days. I should do so well! She only weighs about 100 pounds, so she looks frail, though she is still quite strong.

Homer and Betty came to see Mom last summer and she was having a really bad day. Finally Homer began to moan. "Nobody loves me! I just don't think anybody cares about me at all!" Mom got right up and gave him a hug! Up until that time she had acted completely non-responsive to us!

She also enjoys going for a walk and going for a drive—if I don't drive too fast, and if there's no traffic. I usually drive her out into the country a little.

For Christmas this year, we'll take Mom along when we go to cut a tree. I've already taken her for a drive to look at lights. I'll also take her to the mall and walk her past all the pretty decorations and the children sitting on Santa's lap. These are the kinds of things she can still enjoy. We'll have her out to our home for an hour or two on Christmas Day. She'll be ready to go "home" after that.

If you are receiving this letter, you have been dear to Mom for many years, and I know you would want to know of her. Do send her a Christmas card, perhaps a picture of yourself, or a note. There are occasional sparks of recognition, and she looks at cards and notes again and again.

Love,
Charlotte

I was still able to take Mother on some Christmas outings. She missed cutting a tree because it was just too cold for her to be out. However, there were other things she could do:

I picked Mom up at 5:00 P.M., took her to the mall—about five minutes away by car, and got her home at 7:00. We saw beautiful decorations, many children, and of course, Santa. I couldn't believe how well she walked. I wasn't sure about the escalator but decided to try it once going down. First I asked a young couple if they'd go right ahead of us—in case Mom started to fall. They did, and it was a good thing because she did nearly trip. Of course I had a good hold on her, too. When we had to walk up, we took the stairs, resting every four steps or so. I let her set the pace the whole time. I only let go of her when we were looking at some blankets. Her hands are so busy all the time, but bedding is something soft and safe. We sat down only once for about ten minutes, and she had a glass of lemonade. She's not easy to take to the mall—but once a year isn't so bad!

After I left her, I picked up her picture Christmas cards. I wrote a note to copy and send to each of the people on her list. People say how good I am to do this, but then I think of Magnihild, her cousin who lived on the neighboring farm in South Dakota, and Mable Patterson with whom she went to Norway. These dear souls go back almost eighty years with Mom! Of course they'd like to know how she is from time to time. Both still send notes and pictures to her. How could I not honor that? Many on her list go back fifty years. Some "only" go back thirty. "A person's a person no matter how small." She is still a person, so if I can connect her to friends and relatives once a year—well, it's how I'd like to be treated and how I'd like my friends to be treated.

Some hazel nut brittle was sent to children, grandchildren, Annabelle's Foster Care, and Homer and Betty for Christmas—with the following note:

This hazelnut brittle is one of the favorite treats of The Doctor Agnes, K.E. There is a little farm that I take her to frequently, Kunze Farms, where they grow hazelnuts, a.k.a. filberts. They also grow apples, pumpkins, potatoes, squash, etc., and they keep bees. Some of their things, like filberts, they send away to be made into something wonderful. The finished products they sell in their store along with the fresh produce. It's a rustic, unheated store that is more like a glorified storage shed. Mom loves going in there. When I took her yesterday to pick up the nut brittle, she cheerfully lifted an apple, as she always does, and took a bite. Then she swiped another and took a bite out of it also. I accused her of being a two-fisted thief. The lady at the store knows us by now and laughed at that. They have boxes and boxes of apples in the store, so they never usually even charge us for the ones Mom steals. I always buy Mom some of the nut brittle and then a few things to take back and share with the ladies where she lives.

Anyway, I hope you'll like the nut brittle too. And think fondly of the two-fisted thief who sends it to you!

Charlotte

We had not been able to have The Doctor with us for Easter because we had gone to Poulsbo for a christening in Ralph's family. At Thanksgiving we had friends at our home for dinner, and it would not have been appropriate to have The Doctor there. But our Christmas was small—just Ralph, Janelle and me—so we brought The Doctor home with us to be part of the festivities.

Like I told my good friend, Sharon, on the phone, "Mom's not really hard to take care of now as long as I tie her to a chair." One of the tricks we had learned with The Doctor's agitation was to put an apron on her and tie it around the back of a chair she was sitting in. That way, she could sit still for a few minutes to eat or play with cards or let me go to the bathroom.

Mother had a pork roast dinner with all the trimmings and got a new Cabbage Patch doll from us, a beautiful satin print night shirt from Mary Lou that she kept rubbing against her cheek, and a few other things. Ann had stuffed a stocking for her and each of the other ladies.

The Doctor finished out 1994 weighing in at 98 pounds, fully dressed. Which she rarely was! Once I came into her room, and there she was without a stitch on above the waist. It was getting to be a quality-of-life issue, this taking off her clothes. She couldn't be left in the living room with the other ladies because she'd strip down. Then a husband, niece, or brother would stop in and there would be The Doctor in various stages of undress. Ann had tried jumpsuits, and they did help. It was very difficult, however, to get her in and out of them to go to the bathroom or change a diaper.

Once when I took Mom to the dentist, I had to help her go to the bathroom. I nearly had to wrestle her to the floor to get her out of a jumpsuit. I was sure they could hear us in the waiting room. The Doctor Agnes, K.E., didn't understand what I was doing, so she was not very cooperative.

Thinking about it afterward, I came up with the idea of overalls and found a pattern, some fabric, and a seamstress who would work with us. I explained that instead of hooks for the straps in the front, we needed Velcro *behind* the shoulder where The Doctor couldn't reach it. Instead of buttons or snaps along the sides, a button and Velcro would be easier. I got fabric for four pairs of overalls: light pink corduroy, mint green corduroy, denim blue with a little check, and a beautiful multi-colored corduroy with browns, purples, and hot pinks. We could put on extra pockets and buttons for Mom to play with. By the time we rang in the New Year, the seamstress was at work.

"What is your name? Can you tell me your name?" In a sweet, shy, little girl voice: "Agnes." A big smile and a hug or pat from me. "Yes! And you've practiced that, haven't you?" It was the one thing The Doctor could consistently still do. She could tell someone her name.

Chapter 15

1995

Several sweet letters came after Christmas thanking me for letting them know how The Doctor was doing:

From Gini Pulis, an old friend with South Dakota connections: *Thank you so much for the news about your mother and the photo. I can still see the dear Agnes that I love.*

From Frances Yarrington, whose husband owned the mortuary where The Doctor worked: *It was so nice of you to write and tell me about Agnes. I think of her so often and all the visits and laughs we had. She was always so good to Dick. I get a little lump in my throat when I think about her illness. Doesn't seem quite fair.*

Of course best of all, these and other cards sent to The Doctor decorated her room and occasionally brought forth a glimmer of recognition.

Mom's new overalls were done around the first of the year, and they were adorable. She looked cute and comfy in them, and they made getting her dressed or on the toilet so much easier. Plus she couldn't get them off. I went out and got a few sweaters and turtlenecks for her to wear with them. Tom came in January to visit Mom. He said to her in Norwegian, "Shall we kiss a while?" She puckered right up! They also had a little dance in her room, she in her new pink overalls. Tom thought The Doctor looked better than she had in June. I got some pictures of their dance and even took them to school to show my kids and colleagues.

Even Dr. Laderas commented on how attractive and useful the overalls were. We weighed her in January, and she weighed 104 pounds. By May she was down to 98 again. Not a big loss, but she was so little that every pound was important. She still could feed herself some but often played in her food and had to be fed. Once when I came she had just been served lunch: half a sandwich, lemonade, homemade vegetable beef soup. Mom was hungry, so she tried to lift the bowl of soup to her mouth, but it spilled a little, and she began to cry loudly like a very young child. I dried her off and fed her the rest. She had no problem with appetite most of the time. She ate more than the other people there, when she was eating. Dr. Laderas had checked her thyroid a couple of times, but that wasn't the problem either.

In our state there are trained volunteers—ombudsmen—who come to foster homes to do unannounced inspections to make sure that residents are being well cared for and complying with regulations. There was a new ombudsman who came in January, and he said that Ann was out of compliance because of the Geri-Chair. He said it was a restraint. The tray on the chair had been broken since soon after we'd gotten it. The latch didn't lock. Mom could get out when she put her mind to it. However, it was working so well for the purpose we needed—to focus her eating—that we never bothered to have it fixed. Ann told this to the ombudsman, but he was not satisfied. I got a note and prescription from Dr. Laderas for the chair and had that on file at Ann's. Still the ombudsman was not satisfied.

1-30-95. I went on a retreat this weekend with some ladies from our church. When I got home, I was faced with my relatives from Texas to Anchorage upset over some guy from the state who had been at Ann's on Friday. He wanted Ann to toss out the Geri-Chair—or Mom! Babe happened to call on Friday. Ann told her about it. She called Tom; Tom called John. What a mess. I got everyone calmed down. On Monday (today) I called the guy and told him that we had tried medication for Mom's agitation. It drugged her so that she could hardly walk, and she was so dull. This chair is actually better for her. Ann uses the chair as I'd use a highchair for a baby. I just this week took Mom on a one-and-a-half mile walk. The guy works for the state as an ombudsman, an advocate for the elderly. There's a regulation about restraints. Not so in nursing homes, mind you. In addition, it's perfectly OK in any place to drug people into a stupor. Then I called a woman who worked on licensing foster care homes, Mary Lou Orthman. With the note and prescription from Dr. Laderas and my O.K., she will apply for an "exception to ordinance" from the state for this. So Ann sent the paperwork in, and we'll see what happens—I asked the woman to please advocate for us—I spent about forty minutes on the phone with each of the state people. Heavy sigh.

I had to take a day off work to do this. The state's working hours are the same as mine. It's not as if I can talk on the phone for forty minutes at a stretch with twenty-five second graders around me. I don't even have a phone on my end of the building.

In under two weeks, someone else from licensing came to call at Ann's. This was before a ruling in Olympia could be made on the "exception to ordinance." The new man, James Mead, had an order stating that Mom should be "placed elsewhere."

2-11-95. The translation is that either I move Mom to a nursing home or quit my job and move her in with me! I love it. Mom is perfectly content where she is. The other residents love her. Ann and Ken love her. I, her legal guardian, am happy with her care; her physician is happy with her care. The University of Washington has praised her care. In writing. The state has been sent documentation on all of this and concludes she should be cared for elsewhere! Needless to say, Ann let Mr. Mead have it, and he finally gave in and wrote across the order "No correction at this time."

We still had to wait for the "exception to ordinance," however.

2-13-95. John called today to see how the chair business with Mom is going. I told him that it was hard for me to call these people during my work day. I can't be on the phone with a class of seven- and eight-year-olds. He offered to do the calling and "yell at people" if there's much more trouble, assuring me that he's very

*good at that. It's true. I'll copy all the documentation and send it
to him when the time comes. It's nice to have the back up.*

Another day off work. I was beginning to remember a day in the
hospital as Dad lay dying. He made me promise that I wouldn't allow
Mom's life to be prolonged unnaturally. He told me that all kinds of
pressure would be put on me. I got him to calm down when I assured him
that I was capable of putting up a big enough stink to get my way. He need
not worry. He smiled then, knowing I could do it. Well, it was a different
issue, but the principle was the same. The Doctor was utterly helpless and
at the mercy of others. I was beyond angry.

Every protective instinct in my body was *on fire*.

2-15-95. I spoke with Penny Black in Olympia. [Aging and Adult
Services Administration, Regional Manager and the one with final
say on the "exception to ordinance." Ms. Black had not yet seen
our application for this when I made this call. She had never seen
Mom or her home.] *She told me Mom's exception probably would
not be approved just because they don't like restraints, had seen
many abuses. She further stated that Mom should probably be
placed elsewhere (nursing home) and that I needed to face this.
Never mind that Mom did not need skilled nursing care of any
kind. I blew up at this point and told her that everyone, including
me—Mom's legal guardian, Ann—Mom's caregiver, Mom herself,
Zilpha Haycox, lead psychometrist from the University of Washington, Mom's physician and all of Mom's friends and relatives
were happy with her care. Finally, the cost of her care wasn't
costing anyone but her a single dime. So where does the state get
off saying she has to be in a nursing home?*

*Ms. Black told me to calm down, which I did, and we talked
some more. One thing she explained was that restraints are
allowed in nursing homes because there is 24-hour awake care,
unlike foster homes.*

I got Ms. Black's assurance during that call that my "bad attitude" would not prejudice Mom's application when she did get it. It was clear also to Ms. Black that bad attitude or not, I would never let a denial of the "exception to ordinance" rest. I was fully prepared to call the legislature and the governor if needed.

One of the things Ms. Black wanted was a public health nurse to examine The Doctor. Another call to Mary Lou Orthman in licensing. They had one very trustworthy registered nurse they liked to use in our area. She had been on vacation and that was what was holding up getting the application through. I fully supported this plan. I knew that Mom's care would hold up under any kind of scrutiny. If it did not, I surely needed to know.

Spoke with Marge Meyer (nurse). Marge sounds like a doll. I asked her for a report after she sees Mom.

I also let Marge know that I regularly saw Mom and that I myself had more than once checked Mom's bottom for any sign of bed sores or signs of overuse of the chair.

I called Health Tek Pharmacy and requested that they fix the chair ASAP. It was the only way I could think of to document that the chair wasn't a restraint in the first place because it was broken. The licensing people had this idea that Ann was being "less than forthright" with them. They thought she was lying about the chair, even though she had shown them.

2-16-95. Marge Meyer made a call at Ann's and "inspected" Mom.

2-17-95.
1. Marge Meyer called to say that she found Mom's placement at Ann's appropriate and use of the Geri-Chair appropriate and would report it to Olympia and M.L. Orthman. I requested a copy of the report.
2. I wrote a memo to Penny Black, M.L. Orthman, and Linda Kelley of the Ombudsman's Office defending Ann's integrity and showing the chair had been broken. Mailed copies of memo and

receipt for repair to all.

3. Went to Ann's, cleaned some of Mom's drawers, ran into Linda Kelley and another ombudsman—inspecting at Ann's. Everything looked beautiful, of course.

Now we wait.

It wasn't too long after this that the "exception to ordinance" was approved, allowing The Doctor to stay at Ann's and continue to use the chair.

Several months later, Ann got a questionnaire from the state asking about the ombudsman program. Did she feel it was a worthwhile program? She answered that it was. She felt there needed to be this protection for older people, that there is too much abuse of the elderly, too much potential for abuse without some checks and balances. I'm glad they sent the questionnaire to Ann and not to me. I hadn't cooled down over the incident by then. Still haven't!

Ann got a new lady named May in January. May was very sweet and bedridden.

Ann also was working on training someone new to take a shift at the business. She didn't hesitate to fire someone if she felt they did not keep the place clean enough or attend enough to the residents. When May began to develop a bed sore—something Ann considered inexcusable—the person responsible was immediately fired. Ann trained several helpers before she found one she liked well enough to let her stay alone at "the business." Ann spent more time at "the business" than she did in her own new home, something that was fine with me.

Melissa was a young woman whose father owned a string of foster care homes in the South. Melissa had grown up in this kind of business. She had two children who sometimes came to visit, too.

2-24-95. Melissa's two children (ages three and five) came while I was there. They were going to spend the night and help with preparations for May's birthday party tomorrow. I guess they're putting up streamers and the whole bit...Her whole family is coming for the party, and Ann will have a cake. There were presents there already. I'm sure they were from Ann. Anyway

Mom just lit up when Melissa's children walked in the room! Mom will get dolled up for the party, too. I think she still senses when she looks good.

Melissa added no end of fun to the group. She bought a Richard Simmons workout tape for older people. When she put it in the VCR, Mom immediately got up and got going! Melissa also brought Mom some Legos that she liked to play with.

Melissa came up with the idea of taking The Doctor to a country gospel concert being held at a large church:

. . . a group called The Neelands. She loved it! The look on her face was worth it all. Ralph and I met Melissa there. Melissa had gotten her a new dress, and she looked like a little Easter egg! All bright and pretty. Melissa brought along Fruit Loops and assorted other things to occupy Mom. The Doctor babbled a bit and if the song was really quiet it bothered others. Then we gave her Fruit Loops. However, if it was a foot-stomper, Mom joined right in! We took her home after about 45 minutes, just before intermission. She boogied on out of the place—and nearly stole the show! I saw her again yesterday. Melissa said she'd slept in until 9:30 and had two naps! Still it was fun to do.

I still struggled with the ethics of when to take The Doctor out and where—for a number of reasons. First she was becoming quite frail. So was it best to keep her confined so she wouldn't catch whatever was going around? I didn't feel it would be right to just keep her in for months at a time to protect her from flu and colds. At least to some degree she should get to be out and about. Then there was the issue of her disturbing others. This was kind of like what people think about when they have a baby. I felt it was all right for The Doctor to be in a church to hear The Neelands. But I didn't feel she could be appropriate for a sacred ceremony or a church service. So we no longer took her to church. I especially felt bad about this at Easter. I never got to the point that I was really comfortable with these decisions, no matter which way they went.

Because The Doctor bruised so easily, I joked with Ann that as long as Mom didn't walk around with a black eye, it was O.K. with me. Then one day when I came, Mom had a bruise on her eyelid and another in the corner of her eye!

> *I teased Ann and Melissa about it. Perhaps Mom could have fallen, but the night it happened Ana was in the next room and had checked her every two hours. When we walked today Mom was sharp. I said, "Were you ever a teacher?" "Yes." "Were you ever a mother?" "Yes." "A lawyer?" "No." "A bookkeeper?" "Yes." "Did you fall?" "No."*
>
> *This went on for some time. She indicated "No" at least four times when I asked if she fell. All other answers were correct. She never said "Yes" to the question about a fall. Ann later said she could've just scratched herself, kind of dug at her eye like that. Anyway, it's a mystery. I truly trust Ana, Melissa, and Ann with Mom—and no one else was there.*

Nina never really did recover from the flu in the late fall. She finally quit eating much and passed away peacefully in the winter. She had really grown on everyone. May also passed away in the early spring of '95. Melissa was sitting with her, reading May's Bible to her and singing to her the last few hours of her life.

Without Nina's daughter-in-law, Bonnie, coming to fix the ladies' hair, a new hairdresser was found who would come in. The Doctor got a perm and haircut around the end of March. It took four and a half hours and a bit of misery all around to accomplish the task. We decided that this was The Doctor's last perm.

Weighing Mom was also loads of fun:

> *4-29-95. When we got back from our walk Melissa and I tried to weigh Mom which is quite a job—getting her to put both feet on the scale and not get off when we let go of her. It took about five minutes. Iris [a new resident who had a wheelchair] wheeled herself out of her room to see what the commotion was about. Iris*

is very protective of Mom. She tells me each time I see her how she loves Mom and watches out for her. Mom must know this because every time she passes Iris, she bends down to kiss her or pat on her.

Pearl turned one hundred in June. Of course there was a big party for her. Even *The Columbian*, Vancouver's daily paper, came to Ann's to interview Pearl. Pearl is so sharp. Still a reader and a good conversationalist, she has no patience for The Doctor, however, when The Doctor gets up and stands in front of the TV while Pearl is watching—annoying things like that. Pearl is quite proud of her mind.

Another new lady, named Janet, came. Janet was very demanding, and she lied. She especially lied about The Doctor. Her sister was her guardian, and she believed everything Janet told her. This made both Ann and Melissa furious. They tried to tell the sister that Janet lied about everything, even proved some lies to her. Finally, when Janet told her sister that The Doctor was coming in her room at night, Ken and Ann decided to have a little test. They put The Doctor to bed on the sleeper sofa in the living room. Then Ann and Ken slept on the floor by it. When Janet told her sister again that The Doctor had come in her room, Ken said, "She did not. She slept on the sofa, and she would have had to walk over the top of me to get in there. It didn't happen." Janet didn't last long as a resident.

I was floored that Ken and Ann would go to such lengths to protect Mom. The episode with Janet happened not long after the Geri-Chair business with the state. I called John and told him that it was time to take Ken and Ann out for a treat. He agreed. The four of us went out for dinner at Skamania Lodge, compliments of The Doctor.

Next door to Ann and Ken's new home was another house for sale. They decided to buy it and open another foster care home—right next door. Ann had been having a hard time leaving Mom. She said that when she slept at her own house, she'd wake up worrying about The Doctor. It was because Mom was so totally helpless and because she and Ann were so attached to each other. Ann thought she might move Mom to the new foster care home. I had mixed feelings. On the one hand, no one could care for Mom like Ann. On the other, I hated to move The Doctor. She was frail and very dim. I wasn't sure she should be moved. Tom gave me good advice. He said to let Ann make the call. She was, after all, Mom's primary care giver, and she had proven her love for Mom. I let it rest there.

Ann had a rough spring. Her son, Ken, passed away. Not long after, her brother did, too. She continued work at "the business" while she also was furnishing and setting up the new foster care home. But everything slowed down some because of the personal tragedy Ann was facing.

Then Ken hurt his back and was out of work for a couple of months. All the ladies were happy to have Ken around more. Finally Ann sprained her ankle badly and had to be off of it for about two weeks. She had a cast and crutches. I began to tease the two of them, wondering who was tending whom any more!

Two new residents came. Naomi was also in a wheel chair, a stroke victim. She liked to be babied, but Ann felt she could attain more self-sufficiency. Which she promptly did! There's a bit of an art to taking care of these old folks. Ann had a good sense about when they could care for themselves, when they needed help. She still brushed her teeth *with* The Doctor. She knew how to move people in the right direction.

I sat one afternoon talking with Naomi. I nearly fell off my chair when she said she was raised in Lemmon, South Dakota—same as Mother! That's a very small town. What a small world! Of course Naomi knew some of the names I'd grown up with—Mabel Patterson and her parents, the Jorgensons. She knew others too. Naomi was several years older than Mom, but there were still whole families that both knew.

Hilda also came. She was another who fit in almost immediately.

When Mother's Day rolled around, I selected a fuchsia basket for Mom and all the ladies to enjoy for the summer.

Tom wanted to know what to send—suggesting a doll. I told him I'd gotten her three for 75 cents recently at a garage sale. He suggested sending me 37 ½ cents so we could go in on it together. He can be such a goof. I told him that all the ladies love a treat, suggesting See's candy.

Tom had a box of candy sent to The Doctor and her friends for Mother's Day.

Unfortunately, Melissa left around the beginning of summer. Ann and Ana remained constant, of course. I had visions of Ann spending months again trying to find and train someone new. However, she had an experienced woman named Janice waiting in the wings. Janice worked out very nicely. She was good to the ladies, a great cook, and kept everything in order.

A couple of the ladies liked to watch soap operas on TV in the afternoons. These made The Doctor cry. She could understand that people were not being kind to each other. She couldn't understand that it wasn't real. The news was even worse. It was both sad and real. It shocked and saddened The Doctor to watch it. Other residents wanted to be up on current events. The Doctor was spending more and more time in her little room because she was saddened by what she saw on TV.

Even so, Ann suggested a couple of times that we get a TV for Mom's room. Mom loved to watch old movies with music and dance. She loved the new Western line dancing. Symphony was another pleasure. It amazed me that someone with no mind could have such good taste!

I talked to John about buying one. The TV in the living room had a 35-inch screen. It didn't look like a noisy toy, like a smaller screen might. The close-ups of people were life-sized. It wasn't large and overwhelming like the very large screens. Even without glasses, Mom could see it well. That size seemed about right. John, predictably, told me to go out and get The Doctor a new TV. So when all the Memorial Day sales were on, Ralph and I found and installed a TV. I asked Mom several times if she liked her new TV and got a positive response each time, so I guess she did.

PBS had a documentary on Alzheimer's Disease. The Doctor Agnes, K.E., didn't watch it, but I did. Filmmaker Deborah Hoffman reported both the humor and the joy of caring for her afflicted mother. It was a comfort to me that there was another soul populating this earth who could see this. Perhaps I hadn't gone over the edge after all. Or perhaps we both had.

The Doctor's ability to communicate was one of the hardest things to understand. She might babble for hours on end and then come out with something thoughtful and coherent. I tried to imagine what this brain must be like. Janelle had said like a file cabinet, I had mused about a tape recorder. I sometimes thought maybe it was like a lamp with a frayed wire to it, a bad connection. Sometimes there would be nothing. Sometimes a flicker or a fizz. Sometimes it could light the room.

On a walk in January, amid mumbling that was half words and half nonsense syllables, The Doctor said in her child-like voice, "I have to go poo poo." We went back, and she did!

In February she was sitting with Ken and Ann watching TV. Something came up about Paris.

Ken said, "Agnes, have you ever been to Paris?"

She said, "No, but I've been to Norway." The level of thinking was not merely recall. She was comparing two places. She also knew that Norway and Paris were in the category of Europe. She could have said, "No, but I've been to Sydney" or "No, but I've been to Canada" or Mexico or any number of other places she had been.

In March on a drive I talked to her of Heaven. I had sung "Jesus Loves Me" to her, patted her hand, and told her I hoped it wouldn't be long for her now.

She understood that from the look that came to her briefly knowing eyes.

In March The Doctor could also tell me her name was Agnes, when asked—although not another coherent word came out of her on the same day.

6-17-95. I took her for a long drive in the country, too. She is all babbling anymore, though Ann says she still pops up with coherent words once in a while. She did try to sing with me today—no words just "aaah" with her voice when I was singing "Way Down Upon the Swanee River." She didn't do the tune at all, but it was an unmistakable effort.

Often she greeted Ann with, "Oh, you darling!" She was full of expression, too. We might be out on a drive and come home. When she would see Ann, out would pop. "Oh, you darling!"

One day in July, Ann, The Doctor, and I were in The Doctor's room. Ann and I were talking while Mom sat there just babbling away, not even in words, a steady stream of nonsense. I got nose to nose with The Doctor and said, "Oh babblebabblebabble!"

She laughed, and I could tell by the look in her eyes that she knew I was teasing her about her babbling! It was a rare moment. I asked many times and finally got her to say "Agnes" when asked her name.

Homer and Betty continued to stop and see Mom. They celebrated their 50th wedding anniversary in Seattle in May. Ralph and I went, representing the Leonard family, who had been so close to the Schmitts for so many years.

The Schmitt girls—Susie, Carol, and Janet—gave a wonderful dinner dance for 130 people. It was a lovely event and really honored Homer and Betty. They passed around the mike, so I told a story about how—when going through pictures of their Australia trip with Mom and Dad—I found mostly pictures of the topless beaches. Homer and Dad apparently had quite a time together when they discovered those. I went on to say what faithful friends Homer and Betty had been, continuing to visit Mom—a three-hour drive each way.

I also got to see some old friends. "Bing" Bingham, whose family celebrated Thanksgiving with ours and the Schmitts for over 45 years, asked how The Doctor was doing. I told him that she was content, beautifully tended, and so loved. He said, "What's not to love? Your parents were the most universally loved couple I've ever known."

The Doctor, however, had been having some distinctly unlovable moments throughout the year.

1-7-95. Mom's moods have been changing again lately. She cries, is angry, depressed. Yesterday she spit in Ann's face while Ann was trying to brush her teeth! [Ann would let Mom brush her own teeth and then "touch up" a bit.] *I'll call the doctor and try to get a new Rx for depression. It comes and goes—has for about a month—but is coming more often now.*

1-15-95. I took Mom to the doctor on Thurs. the 11th. She has been increasingly weepy, and I don't need her abusing Ann! We'll try a different antidepressant than desipramine again to see how it works.

1-21-95. I saw Mom last night. She was in the mood to dance! Ken was there, too, putting in a partition in the big room made from the garage. That way they'll have two more private rooms. Anyway it was festive last night with Mom charming us with her dancing. She even did a little jitterbug! Then she went to some fresh flowers on the table and kind of smiled at them. I said, "How pretty! And did someone send those to you?" She patted her hand against her chest. I said, "Yes, my heart would beat fast, too, if someone sent me flowers like that!"

The new medicine gave Mom hives, so she has gone back to desipramine again.

One thing that seemed to happen was that the desipramine would lose its effectiveness. Both Meredith at the U of W and the pharmacist had told me this would happen. So we'd take her off it and try something new. Then when we put her back on it, even after only a short while, it would seem to be effective once again. I didn't really understand it but had observed the same phenomenon several times. This was a medication that worked well off and mostly on for The Doctor for many years.

2-4-94. Ann says the desipramine side effect of the heavy mucous in Mom's mouth seems to be avoided by giving it to her with ice cream. Now Mom gets ice cream morning and night!

This was a worthwhile discovery, allowing The Doctor to have a little higher dose of the desipramine.

Looking back in the journal, many other obvious signs of decline had become evident.

3-17-95. I finally got over my flu and sinus infection so was able to see Mom and take her for a walk...I thought her complexion looked yellow today, but her eyes were O.K. She walked well, too.

3-23-95. Both Melissa and Ann told me that Mom is declining steadily now. I can see it, too. She looks more pale, often sunken and tired-looking. We went for a short walk today. It was really too cold to be out long. She'd spent some time in the yard with Melissa earlier in the day when it was nicer. Mom has done this odd motion that is something between jiggling her body and rocking. She has done it for a few months now. This past week she has been rocking some, too, Melissa said (with no rocker, just rocking her body)—another sign of decline. I've asked her repeatedly if she feels OK, if she hurts, etc., and she lets me know she's fine. It's an odd communication that we have, but I can tell what she means and when our thoughts are connecting.

4-8-95. I saw Mom on Wednesday. I'm getting over a nasty cold—on spring break this week. I'll stop by again today to drop off some cards. Mom still likes to "arrange" cards.

* Took Mom for a drive, and we stopped off at Kunze Farms, where she lifted a couple of apples. The lady there also just put her mother in foster care and is very happy with it. We had a pleasant visit. I bought some honey for Mom to take back to the ladies. Iris's birthday is Saturday. Melissa is having a party for her.*

* Mother's hands were hurting today from her arthritis. She cried out when I was putting on her coat. Then later I took her hands and asked her if they hurt, and she made little crying—whining, mumbly—noises, so I knew that was "yes." I told Melissa to give her aspirin when her hands hurt. Mom's skin tone was yellowish again today for a while—just a tinge.*

4-28-95. Melissa took Mom to the doctor because her hands had turned blue! They were fine by the time I visited her in the evening. The doctor couldn't find the cause, said to watch her and bring her back in a couple of weeks.

6-8-95. I saw Mom yesterday. We went for a drive. I sang everything from "Way Down Upon the Swanee River" to "Jingle Bells."

She likes snappy tunes, the older the better. Beautiful spring day.
She can hardly get in and out of the car any more. Her walk is
increasingly unsteady. Ann said she doesn't think Mom has long
to go now. Twice this past week her face has gone white-pale—
especially white around her mouth—and she kind of sleeps and
then comes to. Iris's son is a fire fighter. He was there once when
it happened. He thought it could be sleep apnea which is a
cessation of breathing during sleep. Ann says also that her feet
turn blue more often. She just rubs them and they "pinken up." One
day this week Mom slept until 10:30 A.M. (Ann changes her diaper
at 5:00 A.M. each morning and then she goes back to sleep.) I do
think Mom is just shutting down.

Along with the decrease in agitation, The Doctor's walk also began to
change remarkably. In January she could still walk a mile or more on a
good day without fatigue. By May, she was often very unsteady. One day
we had an accident that showed me just how frail she was. I took her for a
walk around the block. She wasn't walking well. As we neared home, we
crossed the street, and I stopped at the curb to look at a "For Sale" sign on
a home two houses down from Ann's:

5-18-95. . . . I think she didn't see the curb and kept walking,
although I had stopped. Fortunately I had a hold of her by her left
arm, so it wasn't a hard and fast fall. Her reflexes are non-
existent. She went down in slow motion, one hand still in her
pocket. I had slowly released her other arm as she went down so
she wouldn't wrench it. She fell forward onto the grass, also
fortunate. I lifted her up to a sitting position, and she was crying
child-like, wa-wa. So I said, "Oh, I think you're OK" and gave her
a minute before getting her on her feet. Then we waited another
moment to walk and walked haltingly back. Ann and Ken were
there, so we sat and talked for a while. Mom was favoring her right
arm. Everything else was O.K. She had a chocolate that Tom and
Teri had sent for Mother's Day from Alaska. She may have hurt
her shoulder. Her arm didn't seem broken. I'll call later this

evening to check on her.

*5-28-95. I visited **Mom and took her on a drive.** She was still favoring her right arm, but it was better. Ann kept her quite still and confined for three days after the fall, putting The Doctor's arm in a sling. She's up and around now. Ann still didn't want her to go on a walk yet. She likes to give Mom plenty of time to recover.*

6-1-95. I saw Mom yesterday—took her for a very short walk. She still isn't walking well. Ann says she hasn't danced since her fall, and her arm is still sore. Ann was concerned that the arm wasn't better yet. I called Dr. Laderas this morning and got her in at two o'clock this afternoon—and got a substitute teacher for me, so I could take her. Ann had her all ready to go in a white front-button blouse and her print overalls—very easy to get her in and out of. Dr. Laderas looked at her arm and shoulder. It was still tender near where the collar bone meets the shoulder. However, nothing was out of place. Dr. Laderas said it could be a fracture or a deep bruise. Probably it wouldn't need to be set. Mom would need to have a general anesthetic just to get an X-ray! Dr. Laderas recommended that we just leave it alone and let it heal as it is—especially since Mom has movement in it—though somewhat painful if she lifts her arm.

Realizing just how fragile The Doctor was becoming, Ralph called Meredith at the University of Washington to make sure we had all the arrangements in order for when The Doctor passed away. There would be many details to attend to with the autopsy in another city. For example, Dr. Laderas' records of Mom would have to accompany her body to Seattle. There was no way I wanted to deal with all these arrangements then.

The Doctor did get to the point where she would dance a little again. Not long after this, she did a little dance on the way to the car when we were going for a drive. On other days, though, she was very unsteady on her feet. We only rarely walked around the block after this. A walk of a block or two long was all she could handle. By July, she sometimes staggered when she walked. Once Ken, Ann, and I were in the kitchen with The Doctor. One of the other residents was also there. Ken told me to watch Mother, how carefully she navigated around tables and chairs. He observed that this part of her brain didn't seem to be affected. She was very careful, very precise in her movement. It was true. She wasn't having problems because of things like tripping over things or bumping into something. It was the walk itself that was unsteady.

Ann hired Ana an extra hour a day just to walk with Mom and also take Naomi, who liked being out. Ann wanted to maintain The Doctor's mobility as long as possible.

I continued to take The Doctor on drives, of course, too. On the Fourth of July, Ann was going to barbecue for the ladies, but they became impatient for dinner before Ken got back from the store with the meat, so Ann just fixed them ham and eggs! Naomi's family brought fire works, which The Doctor didn't quite appreciate. I took her for a drive and sang "I'm a Yankee Doodle Dandy" and "You're a Grand Old Flag" as we drove behind a Jeep that had a flag waving. *This* was something she could appreciate!

> *7-24-95. We just went for a drive. Janice, the new gal, seems to be doing fine with Mom. She's a good cook.*
>
> *When we got back, Mom was staggering around the kitchen. I told her she looked like a drunk, and her response told me she understood! She was shocked—jerked back like I'd hit her! So I laughed and said I was just kidding. I asked Janice to make sure that she regularly gets out of her chair.*

Lack of practice wasn't really the problem, though. Ana had reported Mom's hands and elbows turning blue on walks. Then suddenly, The Doctor Agnes, K.E., was sleeping noticeably more.

> *8-1-95. Mom was sitting asleep on the sofa when I arrived. Naomi and Hilda were there, too, watching TV. Mother was stuporous when she woke up. At first I could pass my hands in front of her face with no reaction. It wasn't until she had been awake five minutes or so that she noticed me and smiled. I was sitting right*

next to her, visiting with everyone.

She was a different person from the one who a few months earlier had to be tied into a chair with an apron if she had a cup of coffee at my house! Suddenly, every time she sat for a while, she was falling asleep. The stupor that she had wafted in and out of for the past year also became more common.

The Doctor continued her relentless journey back in time. The careful walk that was staggering, sometimes with arms outstretched, was the walk of someone just learning how. She especially had this look when she got going with the Richard Simmons exercise tapes. The verbalizations that were mostly babble with occasional real words were infantile. Playing with food, needing to be fed. Charming others in an unself-conscious way with a little dance. But what seemed most like a baby was her cry. When she fell, it was the instantaneous "Waaa" of a baby. She stayed down on the ground, too, head down, until I lifted her into a sitting position. She went from being into everything—busy, busy like a child from nine months to two years old—to needing to sleep periodically all day like an infant. Like a baby, she needed tending and love. And like a well-fed, loved infant, she was content.

Of course the *reasons* she was becoming infantile were different from the reasons a baby is infantile. Still, the similarities were remarkable.

Since she could no longer walk to the creek at my house because of the uneven surface of the creek bank, I occasionally took her to the bridge by car and let her look, but it was more often than not lost on her. She wasn't doing well the week before her 79th birthday. We planned to just bring cake and ice cream to her at Ann's and meet Homer and Betty there. I called Homer and Betty a few days before and told them she wasn't doing well. I didn't want them to be shocked. Homer said they'd come down another time. Ralph and I stopped by after lunch with the cake and ice cream. Janice had balloons in the light fixture and a birthday tablecloth on the dining room table. The Doctor sat on the sofa holding a big pink balloon when we came in. The ladies came to the table—Hilda, Pearl, and Iris. Naomi was gone for the weekend with her family. The Doctor smiled as we sang to her. She seemed aware that it was special for her. Afterwards, Ralph and I took her for a drive. She smiled in the front seat at Ralph all the way. When he stopped at Costco, she and I just sat in the car and waited. She fell asleep twice in about fifteen minutes.

I had given The Doctor a large jar of her favorite homemade raspberry jam for her birthday. There was so little she needed. Heather came up with her best gift, I think. She found out how to say "I love you" in Norwegian and taught it to me over the phone from her new home in Boston. I said it to Mom several times with no response at all. Then suddenly, just once, she smiled when I said it, and she knew.

Chapter 16

Turning Points

Somewhere along the line while taking care of The Doctor Agnes, K.E., I had decided that it would never end. For years we had wondered how long this would go on. We had looked at Mom's weight and thought it would end soon. We could look at the rate of decline over a time and decide she wouldn't make it until next Christmas. We watched others at the foster care home come and pass away months or years later, while The Doctor just kept smiling along. Ralph had gotten to the point of saying, "I've guessed wrong so many times, I'm not going to guess any more." So somewhere in the summer of 1995 I grew into a different attitude. I hunkered down and settled with the knowledge that it would go on forever. The challenge would be there as just a part of my life. I used to tell people it was like living with a ticking time bomb in your back pocket. Things would go smoothly for a while and then—*ka-boom!*—off it would go! I'd have to be calling Olympia or running to the doctor or ordering new medications or equipment or clothes. I never knew what would come next, but I knew I was just going to have to live with it. It wasn't going to end.

Ralph's sister, Marilyn, a nurse who had done geriatric work in the past, would hear this kind of resigned edge to me and try to comfort me by saying that it would, indeed, be over one day. Mom would get a cold or the flu, go into pneumonia, and be gone. She said it again at summer's end. I snapped back at her, "Oh, no. Not *my* mother. That may be how the rest of the world makes its exit. But *my* mother will slowly starve to death. Her bones will crumble, and her organs will fail. But she will *not* get sick from a flu or a cold and die of a secondary infection!" Marilyn knew this wasn't easy for me to watch. She was only trying to be comforting.

I had been working on a board in my school district to create a new program for "highly capable learners." The population we were concerned about was that small group, perhaps two per cent, at the high end of academic ability and achievement. Many of these students' needs could not easily be met in the regular classroom. While the district had a one day per week pull-out program for them, there were many reasons why a full-time program would be best for some. This is actually a parallel problem that school districts face with severely handicapped students—those at the opposite end of the spectrum. In both cases it can be argued well to include them in the regular classroom. In both cases, however, there are those for whom this just doesn't work well. After several years of struggling, The Highly Capable Advisory Board—with no little help from parents—was given the go-ahead for a full-time pilot program. I was asked to apply. When I had gone back to work after fifteen years at home, I decided from the start that I would not take on any new challenges until Janelle was through with high school. I extended this to include until The Doctor was gone. Since I'd decided The Doctor would always and forever be around, I was feeling that it was time to get on with my life. I interviewed for the job the second week in August, got it, and immediately swung into high gear. I had to move my classroom to a new school, attend planning sessions and a retreat, and gear up for a new school year with students soon to come from five other schools.

Ann and Ken had started another business, right next door to their new home. Then Ann's brother-in-law passed away, so they had another family funeral—their third in 1995. When Ann was a child, this brother-in-law had come with Ann's sister and taken her and the other siblings out of an orphanage and raised them. It was another big loss for Ann. She had lost her son and brother and now brother-in-law all in the same year.

8-21-95. Stopped in after work. Mom was working on a large plate of homemade lasagna and mixed vegetables. She ate it all, plus two glasses of whole milk. Then we weighed her! She's lost another two or three pounds—was down to 95 pounds fully dressed.

We went over to Kunze Farms. They were busy today. Mom helped herself to an apple and some blackberries. We bought those

and some peaches and took them back for the ladies to share. I
gave Naomi and Iris some blackberries—what a treat!
     We're going to look for a smock for Mom to wear while eating.

While Mom was eating well—often twice as much as the others—she
was becoming less coordinated and messy. Like a young child, though, she
preferred to feed herself and did eat better that way most of the time. It was
when she had something tricky to eat, like soup, or when she had no
appetite that she needed to be fed. Buying her a smock to cover her up
would serve the same purpose as a bib for a baby.

Even though Mom ate well, Dr. Laderas felt that her body was not
using the food well; there was a metabolic disorder undoubtedly from the
effect of Alzheimer's on the brain that was interfering with this function.
From time to time we all wrestled with the fact that The Doctor was
becoming so thin. The alternative was to institutionalize her and put her on
feeding tubes. Beside the fact that her body didn't seem able to use the food
she did eat, this carried the possibility of prolonging her life while simul-
taneously destroying the quality of it. I had promised Dad and Mom's
sister, Babe, that I wouldn't do that. It was not easy watching The Doctor
slowly starve, however.

Janice was doing a fabulous job with The Doctor. Janice was kind,
knowledgeable, and loving. I had thought that no one could replace Ann,
who still came and checked on things regularly, but Janice was remarkable.
Again I marveled at how The Doctor was able to command respect and
love from another human being so late in this disease. Janice fell in love
with The Doctor, always commenting on how loving and good she was.
Janice saw the sense of humor peek through and appreciated the way The
Doctor always patted Naomi when she walked by her wheelchair or leaned
over to give Iris a kiss. The Doctor herself added to a loving atmosphere in
the home. Even though Grandma Pearl was sometimes irritated with The
Doctor, she too recognized the important part Mom played in this home.

Janice had a podiatrist come in to care for the ladies' feet. He clipped
Mom's toenails and removed two corns that had come back. Janice had
worked with the podiatrist before, and this procedure went off without a
hitch. Encouraged by this, Janice decided to try once again to have Mom's

hair permed. This time she washed it the day before to save Mom the trouble of that on the same day. The hairdresser brought some kind of a collar this time that funneled water, so The Doctor Agnes, K.E., didn't have the bother at the sink. The whole operation went much more smoothly, taking only three hours start to finish. The Doctor had an attractive, short cut in the bargain.

There is a demeanor that a young child has when being taken out. It is happy and trusting, ready to go. This was how Mother felt when we went out. She always liked a little walk, a drive, or a stop at the store. Usually when I visited, we'd go out. Perhaps this is why she always greeted my visits with a smile.

> *9-2-95. Saw Mom, and we went for a long drive. It was about 90 degrees out, and she was just right in a sweater and slacks.*
>
> *Janice had gotten her hair permed on Wednesday—short cut, tight perm. It looks really cute.*
>
> *On our drive Mom became suddenly agitated—very! When we got back she had to go to the bathroom right away. The agitation is now her signal for this.*

While The Doctor was incontinent at night, even at this stage she could often communicate this need by day and often went all day without needing a change of her Depends. Of course this required her being watched carefully and continually by the same people who knew her signals. Still, the stereotypical image of someone this far advanced with Alzheimer's is of a person who can no longer walk, who is totally incontinent, and totally unable to communicate. Certainly this was the medical description of the course of this disease. I am convinced that in addition to exceptional care and excellent general health, the fact that we were very careful not to over-medicate The Doctor helped her retain what was left of her abilities. Any sedation at all dimmed this fading and fragile soul. She had only her desipramine at night and as needed occasionally by day.

Research in brain-mapping is something I come across professionally from time to time. Basically the research is telling us that each part of the brain has very specific functions. Perhaps the reason that certain of The

Doctor's faculties remained in place was because the Alzheimer's Disease was not present or was not as severe in some areas of her brain. Control of her bladder might have been an example of this. It is also possible that The Doctor actually re-trained her brain with relationship to keeping the knowledge of her own name. We know, for example, that stroke victims can be re-trained to write, walk, and speak when one area of the brain has been severely damaged. We're told that this is a process of re-routing learning in the brain. When The Doctor sat and practiced her name, was this then the effect it was having? Also I think that general use and ability might help a person retain certain functions. Something a person habitually does, or something a person is exceptionally well-practiced at doing, is more ingrained in the brain. There are more and deeper and interconnected neural pathways with functions that are habitual. This might explain why The Doctor continued to walk at such a late stage of the disease. She was a lifelong walker. A brisk walk was part of her daily routine throughout her life. This also would explain her fascination with cards. They had been a part of her daily life. She and Dad would sit and have a few hands of gin rummy throughout the day. She played bridge regularly. As a child she had learned whist, a form of pinochle that all her Norwegian friends knew. The Doctor's social behavior was also habit. The smile on her face when someone entered her presence was very much a part of her whole life.

At any rate, there were a number of factors that combined to keep parts of The Doctor's personality intact. These included good general health, good care, few medications, ingrained habits, self re-training, and perhaps the sections of the brain less affected by the disease.

The Doctor could also still respond to beauty. She loved a beautiful fall day and often would be out on the deck or in the yard enjoying the sunshine and late-blooming flowers.

In moving my classroom that fall and setting up in a new school, I was running around with a tape measure in my purse. The new TV in Mom's room had been faintly in the back of my mind for some time. It didn't seem to be the same size as the one in the living room. I had specifically bought the same size. However, it was hard to compare sets with them in different parts of the house. So one day on a visit I remembered to measure them and, sure enough, Mom's TV was only a 30-inch TV. I went home and called Ann wondering if she had moved or switched something. But no. I checked my receipt, which said I'd paid for a 35-inch TV. We checked the serial number on the set against the serial number on the warrantee card. They were the same. We had paid for a 35-inch and taken home a 30-inch TV!

9-10-95. Ralph and I went back to Mom's, picked up the TV, and took it to the place we'd bought it. Their computer was down, but they said they'd check their inventory on Monday and call us. [We later got a refund.] *Back to Mom's with the TV.*

When we got back, Mom was having a seizure or stroke. The episode began around 7:00 P.M. on the deck. Mom suddenly got agitated, began to cry and shake her arms, then started to fall. She was seen and caught, put in a nearby wheelchair, and taken to her bed. Her left side was jerking uncontrollably. She couldn't stand or walk, her speech—such as it was—slurred, but she was conscious throughout. We got there then (after she was in bed). The jerking continued off and on. Ana thought we should take Mom to the hospital. Ann and Ken came. They thought we should get a diagnosis and treat it if it was stroke to prevent further strokes and paralysis. They saw it as a quality of life issue. Ralph wanted to take me home.

Ka-boom! Less than two weeks into the school year, the bomb went off again. I struggled to know what to do. Though agitated, The Doctor was not in pain. I was so committed to letting her go when her time came. I hated the thought of the hospital. They would be obligated to run tests, to keep her a while. Away from this home she would be completely lost and confused, unless I was with her every moment. Would she ever get back to these people who loved and tended her? Would she die in a strange place as Dad had? To make matters worse, everyone had an idea about what to do and there wasn't much consensus. "When in doubt, don't." I stalled.

Ann called in a nurse who ran another foster care home. She felt we needed some medical evaluation. Mom's vital signs were good, there was no change in her pupils, and no numbness anywhere—signs of stroke. The jerking continued. The nurse thought perhaps mini-strokes, TIAs. At one point Mom shook her good right arm at Ann and looked fierce about it. Ann said, "I *know* that you're shaking. That's why we're here. We'll take care of you."

The nurse sided with me. We could do nothing, just wait. I would report to Dr. Laderas what was happening. Finally everyone cleared out of Mom's room that night. I waited until she finally went into a rather twitchy sleep before I left her. Ken and Ann brought me home and came in for a short visit. The next day Janice reported that by 6:00 A.M. the jerking had finally stopped.

Before calling Dr. Laderas, I looked back over my literature on Alzheimer's. And there it was—focal seizures at the end of Alzheimer's. My medical book described these seizures as starting on one side of the body, sometimes spreading throughout. Unlike a grand mal seizure that often characterizes epilepsy, the patient remains conscious.

When I called Dr. Laderas, I explained the night we had. She agreed not to treat, but wanted me to report to her regularly.

Of course I also had to report to John, Tom, etc. John was on his way out to sea on a fishing trip but gave me a way to call by way of the Coast Guard. He would call me daily. Tom made some calls to relatives for me.

Tom told me that if I'm ever in the middle of confusion like that again, I should call him for back-up. What a good plan! I have awesome support. I left a message on Homer and Betty's answering machine.

My car has been in the shop all week. I had 150 people at my house for dinner Friday night (a family potluck for the new program I'm piloting). Ralph was in New Jersey Wednesday and Thursday on business. When it rains, it pours.

I went back to see Mom today. She gave me a big smile when I got there! She has some control over her left side. Her mouth was fine (it had been droopy); she could cross her left leg over her right; she could hold a glass in her left hand for just a moment before dropping it. She can stand but not walk yet. She had about two eight-ounce glasses of Ensure. Ana said she'd had a pancake

for breakfast and had eaten a good lunch—needed to be fed. I
asked Mom several times if she had a headache, and she said
"Yes." But she was very happy, peaceful, so I think it was slight.
She kept dozing off and going in and out of stupor. Her eyes were
more sunken than I've ever seen. She was very happy to see me
today—kissy and lovey and peaceful.

By the next day, The Doctor Agnes, K.E., was able to walk slowly. Her balance was off. She was doing even better with her left hand and had the full range of facial expression. She was eating well. Janice said that she was still jerking mildly on the left side from time to time.

On September 13th, Mom walked well enough to get to my car and back, so we went for a drive. It was a beautiful day, and I sang to her as we went along.

Of course I was seeing The Doctor every day. Often I was making phone calls from school to check on things. My work hours became bizarre as a result. I might get to school at 6:00 A.M., or I might be there at 7:30 P.M. Or I might be there on a Sunday afternoon. I saw Mom sometimes before school, sometimes after. Sometimes I saw her between school and a meeting. I just was squeezing things in whenever I could. Ralph's job had taken him out of town almost constantly in 1995—and at this point it seemed a blessing.

The Doctor continued to have the focal seizures off and on. The best way I can describe them might be to borrow a slang phrase from childhood —"a *spaz* attack." She was alert but not in control.

9-15-95. I went after school and Mom was worse still. Very
agitated and having spasms on both sides—not just the left. She
can't stand and has somehow hurt her left hip. She cries out when
she moves at the joint, though she can move from the knee down
with her jerking and has no pain there. She keeps trying to sit up
and then cries out in pain. Then she forgets and tries again. It's
pitiful.

There is a time for sedation and that time has come. I called
Dr. Laderas at home, and we got a prescription. Dr. Laderas

reconfirmed my wishes on the DNR order. When the first dose of medicine wasn't enough to calm Mom, we gave her another. I do want her kept comfortable. I left when she finally was dozing...

Janice is the best. She understands and agrees and supports letting Mom go. Ann understands this and agrees on an intellectual level, but emotionally her instinct is to treat. She keeps wondering why Dr. Laderas doesn't put Mom on this or that. It's because we don't want to fix Mom and make her well enough to be a vegetable for the rest of her life. Ann understands and tries, but it's like it goes against who she is. I can't fault her for it. I'm grateful Janice is here, too.

9-16-95. Janice called this morning with the news that Mom was much worse. The seizures are affecting breathing. I had both school and house work to deal with but rushed to get over there.

Here I sit. Mom is awful. She sort of chokes, breathes, stops breathing. It's noisy and grotesque. Frightening to her and me. I've put Vaseline on her mouth which is so dry from breathing with her mouth open. Janice showed me how to use a straw to deliver drops of water to the side of her mouth. It scares me. She has so little control I think she'll drown. She dozes off and on. I fed her ice cream. She does better with that. I'm freezing Ensure to try on her.

Still, she had a big smile for me today once when she "clicked in." She doesn't really talk but can make sounds. It scares her when she can't breathe—which is every few minutes. So I tell her it's OK—it only lasts a moment. She hasn't turned blue or anything. Her color is good.

Ralph went to Health Tek and brought in a hospital bed, so we can move her upright without hurting her hip. This helped her greatly. They don't deliver on weekends, and we didn't want to wait until Monday to make her comfortable.

Having the hospital bed also helped keep her upright to breathe. When not in a stupor or very agitated from the shaking, The Doctor continued to smile through all of this. She would kind of awaken from her stupor, see one of us, and give us that beautiful smile. The books all said that Alzheimer's patients lose the ability to smile. But not The Doctor. Ralph said it was just the way God made her.

Because I wanted someone with Mom every moment when she was having a hard time, I made a deal with Ana to come over on an on-call basis. She kept track of the hours, and I paid her for it. It was too much to expect Janice to take care of four other ladies and be with The Doctor all the time, too. It really comforted Mom to have someone there.

John offered to come when Ralph left for a business trip to help, but I was looking forward to a little solitude, and by the time Ralph left, things were at least momentarily stable. However, it was comforting to have John on stand-by. He could be here in just a couple of hours by plane.

Ann was also coming over about twice a day to check on The Doctor. Since the last seizure episode, Mom had not walked. It was hard for Ann to see Mom bedridden. I had to get a new supply of this and that to accommodate a new lifestyle for Mom. She needed a couple of dusters that snap in the front to wear in bed. Janice needed some new toiletry items to keep The Doctor comfortable.

As September 19th approached, the fourth anniversary of Dad's death, I remembered all the times The Doctor had said when she worked at Yarrington's that someone had died on or near a milestone day. It happened far too frequently, she believed, to be coincidence. They most often died on or very near their own birthdays. Sometimes it was another milestone day, perhaps a mother's birthday, an anniversary, or some other important event. She would wonder if this were some kind of a biological clock, or perhaps it was celestially caused. At any rate, this came back to me as September 19th approached. I had always said that The Doctor and Dad were joined at the hip.

9-18-95. Stopped off at Health Tek on my way over. Got swabs for the inside of Mom's mouth.

She was better today. Had cereal for breakfast, spaghetti for lunch. I fed her a bowl of finely chopped chicken, broccoli, and rice plus an eight-ounce glass of frozen Ensure! Toward the end

*she'd fall asleep with her mouth full! (then woke up) Brushed her
teeth.*

*She's currently into old Shirley Temple movies—waves her arm
at the TV if we try to turn it off! It has seemed to comfort her the
past few days.*

Seizures have stopped again now.

*I think her left eye is infected. Talked to Home Health
nurse—one coming tomorrow to check on her.*

*When I left, I gave The Doctor a kiss and said, "No wild
parties now!" She said, "I love it!" She was sharp today—told me
"Agnes" the first time I asked her name. She was able to breathe
with closed mouth today and sleep.*

The nurse came the following day. After she raved about Mom's wonderful care, she said she didn't know why The Doctor wasn't walking. The
pain has subsided, but The Doctor is completely content to be in bed. The
nurse wondered again about the possibility of stroke. I still felt it was focal
seizures we were seeing. These came and went, leaving a temporary stiff-
ness or drooping in affected areas. The Doctor's mouth drooped, while her
hands became stiff. Sometimes in the last couple of days they had seemed
to close her throat. That's why she needed someone with her to tell her
each time that this only would last a few seconds. She couldn't remember,
but she did understand when told. Again I pointed out that stroke is marked
by numbness and lack of movement. We'd had pain and constant moving.

In fact, The Doctor was the most hyperactive bedridden patient I'd ever
seen! I'd come to visit, and there she'd be with one skinny leg flung over
her bed rail and the bedclothes all messed up. She'd have cards and toys
and her baby all over the place, and Shirley Temple singing and dancing on
the tube. So I'd fix The Doctor Agnes, K.E., up. I'd tidy her bed, arrange
her toys, straighten her duster, tuck her leg back in and tuck in the
bedclothes. Three minutes later, there she'd be with her leg flung over the
bed rail, cards strewn here and there, pillow out of its case, sheets rumpled
in a corner. She was so busy!

The nurse told us that we could have a special machine brought in to
X-ray Mom's hip. A good idea.

9-19-95. . . . I'm sooo tired of this. So detached feeling, unemotional, ready for it to be over.

Janice had seen Mom take her doll's bottle and suck on it. We didn't know if she was trying to communicate that she was thirsty, or if she was delusional and thinking this was a real bottle. At any rate, I had a small baby bottle at home that I brought over. Sure enough, The Doctor drank from it. It was a way to make liquids readily available to her.

Fortunately there were some genuinely happy things going on around me. I needed that balance. Janice's cat had kittens. Six—five of them Manx, without tails—and one with a tail. I would bring one in to The Doctor and rub it softly against her cheek. My journal recorded their growth, such a bright spot were they for me:

Two kittens had their eyes open today.

My own family also was a diversion, though not always a happy one. Janelle had gotten pneumonia the same week my school was starting. The whole family was in panic over it. She'd also blown out an eardrum with a sinus and ear infection, was supposed to be moving from her summer home back onto campus at the University of Rochester. It was a mess. Heather ended up renting a car after work one day and driving from Boston to Rochester, arriving at 1:00 A.M. and tending to her sister. Heather moved Janelle, fed her homemade chicken soup, and stayed until Janelle was out of trouble. Considering that Heather was getting ready to start graduate school and still kept her job in the International Scholar's Office at M.I.T., the trip was a sacrifice for her, too.

Janelle was also upset because she needed ensemble work for her music major and couldn't audition on her French horn, her secondary instrument, without functioning lungs and with a ruptured eardrum. Of course we told her that her first job was to get well.

When she was well, the ensemble auditions were over. However, she found out that there were some vocal ensembles that would also meet the requirements. So she auditioned for a choir and made it in based on her "good ear." We had a big laugh over that.

My journal entry for September 22nd:

Carnegie Hall!

I didn't have time to write the rest, but it stood alone as a reminder that amid all the craziness with Granny, there was this joy. The choir Janelle had gotten into had been in a choir competition in Wales the previous summer and had done very well. Two weeks into the school year they were asked to open a choir concert in Carnegie Hall in June! Ralph also took time when he was in New Jersey to rent a car and drive to Rochester to make sure Janelle was really healing well.

Meanwhile, The Doctor stabilized some while Ralph was back East again. She had broken her hip, the x-ray revealed. This put to rest the idea of a stroke. The break was near the pubic bone. It was probably a spontaneous break. The nurse said that for her to have bumped it in the place near the break, she would have had to be doing the splits! Undoubtedly someone would have noticed. It could have broken during a seizure, or it could have just broken on its own. The Doctor was so very thin. Although it wasn't possible to weigh her on a bathroom scale, we knew she had lost more weight because the eating would go when the seizure activity was high. Then she'd eat constantly when it subsided.

A special mattress was brought in that inflated in various areas over time, relieving pressure to any one area. This was used to prevent bedsores. Mother was also turned regularly and would chatter along incoherently even as she faced the wall.

I really was struggling with the idea—again—of letting The Doctor go naturally. With the hip broken and the seizures causing uncontrollable movement, it seemed impossible to both keep her comfortable and let her go. Ralph pointed out that between the weight loss and the seizures, she could break every bone in her body one by one. So I approved, finally, of some seizure medication, so the hip could heal, and so she wouldn't break more bones with seizures. While the break was such that it would never heal, so she could walk without surgery, it could heal to the point of not being painful. Indeed, The Doctor was able to sit sometimes in her Geri-Chair after a few days to play with her cards and watch TV from there. She could also stand without pain and with a little help for just a moment—getting from chair to bed, for example.

The Home Health Nurses had a new and improved DNR form for me to fill out and sign. I loved having a little more paperwork to do. In my journal I'd call it a day off if I "only" went to work and ran my own household. But there was to be only one of those for a long while.

9-23-95. Tom called. He'd asked a doctor friend of his about Mom. The guy said if it was his mom he'd withhold food and water for 36 hours, at which point she'd go into a coma and die. I pointed out that doing something to cause death is called murder—and I have to live with myself when this is over. Did he want to come down and do this?

Of course he didn't, and he hadn't really thought this through. He certainly hadn't intended to rile me! However, this gives an idea of what people—if they're honest—go through and think about. Tom's *intention* was to relieve suffering—Mom's, mine, and his. And I knew that.

Zilpha Haycox came down from the University of Washington to see me and check in on Mom. To mentally prepare herself, Zilpha had decided in advance that The Doctor was dying and would be non-responsive and withdrawn. The Doctor was quite sleepy and expressionless at first. I wondered if it was from the seizure meds that she had just started. But Zilpha was surprised by the way Mom came to life when I came in. She was still very much alive, smiling and responsive. Zilpha felt Mom got her energy from me. Of course I'd seen her light up like that with Ann and Janice, too. The Doctor was still quite social. This was another of those ingrained habits of hers. She was not only still able to reach out to people, she was able to win their love and affection. Janice and her son Joshua had only been in Mom's foster care home a few months; both were devoted to her. When we left, I put my cheek next to The Doctor and asked for a kiss, which I promptly got.

After Zilpha went on her way, I went to Health Tek to pick up a new prescription for The Doctor's stubborn eye infection and some wipes that Attends puts out for adults.

9-24-95. Well, I lost that detached feeling today. Finally made it to church for the first time in three weeks, knowing I needed to be filled up, suited up for the week ahead. The vocalist sang "It Is Well With My Soul," and I started to cry. It's 6:15 P.M. right now. I've had a nap, but still the tears keep coming. Time to let Maisie (our dog) take me for a walk. Many people praying for Mom and me now.

Speaking of prayer, I'd thanked God for Dr. Laderas more than a few times in the past years. She was such a good listener, careful to help in the way Mom, Dad, and I needed help. I'd wanted for a long time for Dr. Laderas to visit the foster care home. I had Dr. Laderas' home phone number and had to call her a couple of times. Over the weekend she had told me that she really felt she should see Mom. With the broken hip, I would have to get an ambulance to take Mom there. When Dr. Laderas suggested that she visit Mom at the foster care home, I volunteered to pick her up and take her there myself.

9-26-95. I picked Dr. Laderas up at her office and took her to see Mom. Of course she was impressed. She stayed an hour and twenty minutes. I fed Mom a big dinner—cottage cheese and peaches, broccoli, mixed vegetables, chicken with mushrooms and stuffing, and fettuccine. Then Mom had an ice cream bar! No one can believe how much Mom eats. Dr. Laderas asked for Ann's card and on the way back raved about how pretty, clean, and homey it was. She even had a look at the kittens. Dr. Laderas lives with her 91-year-old father. She also praised Janice. Ann and Ken stopped by—I had told Ann Dr. Laderas was coming.

Mom looked good enough to last another year.

I'm too tired to think about it.

The seizure medication brought a stability to The Doctor's life. However, she had times when she really did not look good. Her complexion would be gray. Often when she slept, the skin around her mouth would be white. Both were indications of a lack of oxygen. While she never had a fever or congestion, her breathing was labored off and on. She just sounded and looked like breathing was work. Then it would go away. She was being checked every couple of days by a nurse, so we knew she didn't have pneumonia. There was one time that Janice had to work to wake The Doctor in the morning. I told her not to do that again. A little more time, perhaps, and The Doctor could go into a coma and slip away peacefully.

Once when Janice was turning The Doctor while I was there, The Doctor cried out. I asked Janice if Mom was still in pain. She said no, Mom just didn't like to be moved. It startled her. Janice told me to watch. Janice put her face in Mom's and said quite firmly, "I am going to move you that way," at which time she pointed to the wall. Then she turned Mom and Mom did nothing more than make little "oh, all right" noises. So she wasn't in pain just then, and she could still understand—even on the pain meds—when her attention was focused.

10-3-95. Big smile when I came in. "Not good, but I'm beautiful" is what Mom said when Janice asked her how she was today.

"Agnes Leonard" she said the first time I asked her name. "Yes" three times when asked if she hurt. Janice had been having problems again with Mom not sleeping at night. We may need more again for pain. The hip is bothering her again. She expresses it by rubbing it, by rocking back and forth. Perhaps by not sleeping well at night.

Color was good today. She thought I was "beautiful." A much better day. Kissy again.

My boss told me to be sure I'd said what I had to say to her. So I told her how loved she is and how forgiven. I told her of her children. Sadness was on her face when I told her that her old South Dakota friend, Mabel Patterson, had just died. I told her it was her turn.

I'm angry inside that she and I have to keep going through this. I hate her being bedridden.

I was very angry at God at this point. I had specifically prayed for years that The Doctor would always be able to walk. Of course God is not Santa

Claus. And we can't control Him by our prayers. But logic wasn't my strong suit at this time. I was just angry at having to watch someone so innocent and loving, so dependent and helpless, so active and busy be confined to bed. It felt like watching a crippled child. She could not understand her situation.

Back on my own home-front, Ralph was being honored for some work his team had done—a weekend in Las Vegas that could include spouses. I put off deciding if I could go until just a few days before the trip. Finally, I decided to go along. The Doctor was relatively stable. We had a wonderful time. I'm not a gambler, but there was plenty to see and do for our three days there, and it was a real break for me.

When I got back, I again wrestled with the ethics of Mom's situation.

10-15-95. By treating the seizures have I sentenced her to a longer life bedridden? The hip will probably never heal. Should I have had her put on morphine and let the seizures continue? I didn't know at the time this was an option. (Janice just told me. We had been talking about the difference between Hospice and Home Health Nurses. I'd been given the option, but when I asked what the difference was, no one had told me that with Hospice we would just get "comfort care" and let her go. I had been told that Hospice was for the end of life at which point I'd said something like, "And how can you tell? We've thought Mom was at the end of life for years!" So she had been put with Home Health Nurses.) There's no easy way.

Again I wrestled with God. And with myself. Who was I to think I could have any say in the timing of Mother's death? Did I think I could control *life*? What arrogance on my part! All along I had struggled to let God be God—sometimes at the point of saying to Him, "So *be* God, then! Do *something!*" I also wondered: at what point do we become the hands of God? I generated far more questions than answers.

There was a comfort in going through this with others. I tended to visit when I was the only visitor—early mornings or evenings. Now that I was there midday on weekends, too, I saw other visitors more often, and this was uplifting to me.

Naomi's family also visits with Mom when they come, much as I stop and visit with Naomi and the others when I come.

Visiting briefly with Iris's son or Naomi's daughter gave me a perspective that I was not the only person on earth with these responsibilities. I have a close friend whose child has multiple, life-threatening handicaps. Another friend, not much older than myself, is in a nursing home with multiple sclerosis. These ties also served to give me badly needed perspective.

Meanwhile the higher doses of pain medications caused constipation for The Doctor, which necessitated *more* medications, as is so often the case. It made me glad we hadn't had a lot of medications earlier. They just seemed to complicate things. The Doctor's appetite decreased again.

I tried to feed her, but except for two helpings of ice cream, it was no-go. Janice came in and broke up her food into little pieces and Mom ate it with her hands. Her coordination isn't very good any more to eat with utensils, but she could eat with her hands, baby-style—and she did!

I have been feeling detached from The Doctor lately. I fight it because I don't want her to feel she is dying alone. I know she still feels what others feel around her. She is playful with Janice from time to time. This week she held onto Janice and laughed and squeezed tighter when Janice tried to let go of her. Occasionally she'll be lucid, telling Janice once last week to "be careful" when Janice turned her. Also she told Janice to "Come, come, come!" when she saw an ice cream bar in Janice's hands. Still, since the seizures it has been hard for me to be happy when I hear she's eating well. I feel it's time for her to go. I feel emotionally spent.

When I found out that we could have put her on morphine and let her go that way instead of treating the seizures I've felt guilty. That would have been the right way to go. I wasn't told it was an option.

A close friend, Ron Detrick, called about this time, giving me a chance to talk this through with him. He asked what was stopping me from taking her off the seizure medications and putting her on morphine now. This is the same ethical issue families face when deciding to take a person off feeding tubes, IVs, and other forms of life support. It feels like *causing* death. It's so much easier not to have them on these things in the first place. It took me a while to think this through and realize that it would be the *seizures* that were causing death (or lack of ability to eat, breathe, and so on). I would simply be allowing that to happen by removing the medicine. Still, to do that would require some support. I did not want to offend the people who lovingly cared for Mom. Ana, Ann, and Janice had literally been up nights caring for The Doctor. They could at any time say it was too much, that we needed to move Mom. I wanted to be careful of their feelings in this. So I talked about it with each of them. It took me a week after talking to Ron to come to this. They also needed time to think. I just wanted to begin to build consensus. I wanted to raise the possibility that if the seizures began again, because she was on a very low dosage of the medication, I might choose a different course.

The talk with Ron also let me know that I wasn't as emotionally detached as I had thought I was. I was still completely capable of being very emotional and protective of The Doctor.

Having settled this within myself, I caught a cold. Within forty-eight hours I had bronchitis and an ear infection! I was effectively grounded from school and The Doctor. However, it gave me time to come up with a thank-you gift to Janice, Ana, and Ann. I told John and Tom that these three had gone way beyond the call of duty all fall on The Doctor's behalf. They needed a little treat. We got them each gift certificates for their families to spend a weekend at the beach.

10-23-95. The kittens are nearly grown now. Naomi's daughter is taking four of them for barn cats. The other two have been given away. The ladies have loved watching the kittens through the sliding glass door to the deck off the dining room.

Iris would wheel her chair right up to the glass door and sit there and watch the kittens. They were a delight. The kitten who had a tail had to put up with the whole group chasing hers, since the others had no tails. It was a riot. The weather was too cold for the ladies to go out, but Janice had the kittens' bed and food right outside the door for the ladies to watch. Of course all the visitors also had to spend some time with the kittens.

There's a kinship that develops among those of us who come to visit our mothers. We each visit with the others besides our own. We each respect one another for this place we're in for our loved ones. Hilda's son came as I was going last time. He also checks on Mom.

We're so fortunate to have such kind and dedicated souls caring for Mom. It makes my life livable. Part of why they do it is that Mom continues to give so much back. She kisses and hugs them, sometimes still says, "Oh, God, I love you!" when they help her.

Mom's smile, while usually soft and warm, sometimes had a haunted look to it. That had been so for perhaps two years on an occasional basis. Tom noticed it on his last visit. It was more common in the last six months. Still her beautiful smile peeked through daily. She told Janice one day she was Agnes Leonard through a mouthful of food. Knowing her name and keeping a smile on her face were the two things she had worked on keeping. It was her own personal triumph to keep these little things. We who loved her to the end had a profound respect for the courage, tenacity, and fierceness that she mustered to accomplish this. She had precious little else, but *this* was dignity.

If I've learned nothing else with all of this, I've learned that somehow The Doctor herself remains. She still can say "yes" if I ask her if she's hurting. Beyond this primitive kind of awareness, Mom is there—a lady or girl or child who loves to be told she is pretty, who smiles at this. A person who is loving and affectionate. A very busy person who plays at her cards still, moves constantly, flinging her leg over a rail, exercising her arms, legs, and body all the time. A person with a sense of humor who likes to play. A woman with good taste in music and dance, who prefers this to soap operas on TV. I thought she would be "gone" by now. I hear people say things like, "She's not really there" in response to the fact that she can't call me by name. But she is really there. And she does know who I am, though she can't put a name on me or on our relationship. I can see it by her expression every time that I come.

It is by her own will that she keeps a smile on her face, by her own will that she remembers her name, by her own will that she keeps on loving. Her dignity seems to transcend all loss of ability. It comes from something quite apart from that.

I was having bad dreams before I talked to Ron. One was where there was nothing left of Mom but her head flopping around. Her body had shriveled up, leaving only her head with sad eyes.

The dreams have stopped now. I feel right about the decisions made. The guilt is subsiding. Sometimes there's no right way, and a person just does the best he or she can do then and must live with that.

11-4-95. What a wild week it has been! I went back to school healthy at last. On Monday, the 30th Mom woke up having obviously had seizure activity. She couldn't make intelligible speech, barely used her right hand, and was in some pain. Eating was altered because of difficulty chewing and swallowing. She was eating pudding, Ensure, ice cream, and taking fluids administered by slowly emptying a needle-less syringe into the side of her mouth. I saw Mom before school Monday.

The nurse came later, and I spoke to her by phone from school saying that it was time to let Mom go; she needed to call Hospice. So Hospice was called—probably on Tuesday—but they didn't come till Thursday. Anyway, I called Dr. Laderas Monday after work, and she told me that she'd talked to the nurse and upped the seizure medication! I said no, I wanted—if anything—to remove seizure meds when Mom went onto morphine. I wanted to let her go. Dr. Laderas agreed. I told her Hospice would be in touch.

Tuesday. I saw Mom after work. She was slightly worse. I didn't stay long. Halloween.

Wednesday. I saw Mom after work. She was eating even less, color was not as good. I had a meeting that ended early so spent the late afternoon and evening.

Thursday. Another afternoon meeting, so I was able to break away early. The Hospice folks showed up, so we got papers signed, and they got the background and let me know of their many services. They offered social workers and grief counseling, nurses, volunteers that will sit with the patient, clergy for spiritual counseling. I have a solid support group in Janice, Ana, Ann, Ken, Ralph, Heather and Janelle, my church friends, boss, brothers, the teacher I team with, my other teacher friends and staff at my old school, Hearthwood, and the folks at the U of W who have seen me through all of this. So I don't really need a social worker. My friends from church have done plenty of praying for and with me. Our pastor is a personal friend. I don't really need clergy either. What I needed and wanted was to get Mom more comfortable and on morphine. Since Monday she had been asleep, wafting in and out of consciousness—only awake perhaps an hour or two per day. They asked if it could wait till morning or if I wanted it now. I asked the nurse and Janice what they thought, and all agreed that morning would be fine. But at 1:30 A.M. Mom started having more seizures and some pain. Janice gave her extra pain meds and sat with her the rest of the night.

One day when I came to visit, Ana was in the front, sweeping the walk. She was crying. Such a dear lady, so good to The Doctor. She was crying because she knew we were near the end. When Ana worked, she sometimes had her children with her in the evenings and overnight. Her children would come into Mom's room when she was attending Mom. Her youngest daughter would play on the floor at the foot of Mom's bed. This was really a part of Mom's family. These children loved her and were comfortable with her, whatever state she was in. Likewise, Janice's teenage son, Joshua, would stop in Mom's room a few times each day, just to check on her. He was very sweet and cared very much about how Mom was doing.

The journey back for The Doctor was now complete. She was an infant in nearly every way. She drank sometimes from a bottle, needed to be fed. All of her needs were met by others. She could communicate in only a very primitive way, except that she knew her name. And so it was that while The Doctor Agnes, K.E., never really did know everything, she always managed to know *some*thing!

11-3-95. By now I was calling in multiple times a day. So when I got the call at school at 10:30 to come, it was no surprise. Mom's color had gotten very bad, breathing very labored, her nails turned black. Fortunately, my boss was next door in my partner's room, and she came in and took over for me. By the time I got there, Mom's nails were OK, but she was obviously working to breathe. She'd had no food or water.

The Hospice nurse arrived and we started Mom on the morphine. She wanted to see Mom's respiration lowered to twenty per minute or less (it was twenty-eight) and less labored breathing. It took a while to get that consistently, and it wasn't until 4:00 P.M. perhaps that it was under steady control. A catheter was put in, so Janice wouldn't have to move Mom so much to change her. I stayed on, helping myself to the kitchen as needed. Ralph came and took me out for a while for dinner. Then around 7-7:30 P.M. I began to notice that Mom's breathing was slowing. It went from eighteen to fourteen to twelve to eleven. It stayed at around eleven for a couple of hours. It was now after 9:00 P.M. Ana came in. I had cleaned and lotioned Mom's mouth a couple of times. She was unresponsive. I told Ana to watch mom while I turned on the ceiling light. Earlier in the day she had winced at that. This time there was no response. She was in a coma. Now we could close her eyes, and they stayed closed. I went home finally.

This is also hard on the ladies who live with Mom. It puts a cloud over the home. Although I am cheerful around them, it's still hard on them. The kittens provide the comic relief. One kitten, the cutest actually, has a nerve problem with one back leg and is handicapped. She hops like a rabbit. She's adorable and fluffy, though, and all the kittens have a home they're going to.

Friday night when I got home I called John and Tom. Janelle called. Then I went to bed.

Saturday. By Saturday morning Mom's breathing was slower yet. For three hours in the night it had slowed to three per minute. By morning it was six to eight, irregular, and often very shallow. Now one had to look hard to discern breathing.

The nurse had said that sometimes patients will finally relax when put on morphine and let go and go into a coma. She didn't think Mom would do that, though, since her vital signs were so strong. Still she noted that because Mom was so very emaciated, there wasn't any reserve left.

I spent a couple of hours Saturday morning "being a person" before going over. I just needed to sweep a floor, take a shower, drink my coffee, play some solitaire. I called Janelle and Heather, Babe, Homer and Betty, my boss. I called a message into my students on "The Classroom Connection."

So here I sit. I check mom's respiration, clean her mouth with wet sponges, put Vaseline on her lips. And wait. I'm actually getting good at waiting.

At school this week I was forgetful and ditsy. I told a friend from my old school, Hearthwood, that it's hard going through this at a new school where no one knows me. They think I'm always like this!

11:40 A.M. Sat. Still I've had the strength to do things I didn't think I could do. I've been able to sing hymns to Mom a little. I thought I would just cry. I took her off all seizure medication after we started the morphine. She started having seizures a few minutes ago. This brought her into an agitated semi-consciousness again. Her eyes are very cloudy and sorry-looking. She has them half-opened, and she blinks, which makes me think she is somewhat conscious, so I talk to her. There's a very fine line here between consciousness and the lack of it.

11-5-95. Another long day. Mom had a fever of 102.7 degrees—a sign of dehydration, the Hospice nurse said. We got her quite a bit cooler and her temperature down by removing some covers and changing her duster. Still no sign of lung congestion. The Hospice nurse turned Mom and checked her catheter. This little bit of movement sent Mom back into labored breathing that stayed the same and regular the rest of the day. Seizure activity increased. Just uncovering Mom's hands to look at her circulation seemed to set off small seizures. Because of the seizures Mom was semi-comatose, the nurse said. Mom could blink her eyes and suck on a sponge to cool her mouth.

This day was a rough one. Midday I left Mom and went over to school to get my classroom in order. Between my illness and now this, my class was falling apart. I did what I could to prepare plans for the following week, then went back and stayed with The Doctor until late evening. When I finally got home I told Ralph two things. First, I could not continue like this. I had to do one thing or the other. I would have to temporarily leave my class. I arranged for my favorite substitute to come in Monday morning to take over. Second, no matter what happened, I needed to be at school Monday morning! While this seemed a contradiction, I needed to calm my students. My boss had told me that Friday afternoon had been a mess. I needed to bring in some order, even model for the substitute how tight I wanted the ship run for a while.

For two months I had been exhausted with the care of The Doctor. However, like the last days spent with Dad, I would not have chosen a different way. It is a sacred honor to be near a person who is dying. It is a sacred trust. Tired was a price worth paying.

11-6-95. Janice called at 4:30 A.M. Mom had given an audible little sigh and stopped breathing. She was gone. Her heart contin-ued to beat, however, for some time.

It had perplexed Janice so much that she had run over to Ana's house in her bathrobe and knocked on her window to awaken her. Ana had come over to confirm that The Doctor was gone—though her heart was still beating. Janice then called me.

Ralph and I drove over. The Doctor's body was still warm, her eyes still open. She was on her mattress that inflated and deflated to change pressure points. Perhaps because that was turned on, it seemed that there was still motion in her body. We turned it off. I closed The Doctor's eyes. They opened again. A few minutes later I closed them again, and this time they stayed closed. Her heart had also stopped beating.

It was the day before what would have been her fifty-third wedding anniversary.

My concept of death forever changed. Perhaps it is the influence of TV that makes us think that death occurs when the heart stops beating. But Dad's heart stopped beating for some time before he died. I know this is so because he was talking to me and John after three nurses had spent some time trying to find a pulse. The Doctor's heart beat for some time after she was no longer breathing. I no longer think the beating of a heart in and of itself as a sign of life or death. Again perhaps because of TV, we think of death as occurring in an instant. I no longer believe that either. I think it is more accurate to say that it occurs in a moment—and that moment may be a short one or a long one. I do know that for the rest of Monday, even when I came back later in the afternoon, there was a sweet peace in The Doctor's room that was pervasive. I'll never forget it.

The Hospice nurse arrived by around 5:30 A.M. and listed Alzheimer's as the cause of death. The mortician arrived soon after and took away The Doctor's body. Then Ralph and I went out for breakfast, more to talk things over than to eat. After that, I went to school and set my class in order, telling them that I would be gone for the week to finish the funeral and so forth.

I wonder what it will be like to have my life back?

Chapter 17

Going On

The next week, I did some finishing-up things at the foster care home. I delivered the gift certificates, cleaned out The Doctor's room, wrote a letter of recommendation for Janice, and updated a similar letter for Ann. I left some of The Doctor's clothes for the ladies. When I gave Hilda a pink sweater because she said she was cold one afternoon, she thought I'd given her quite a prize.

John was in Seattle right away making arrangements there. Mom had always wanted to be buried, while Dad had wanted cremation. After Dad's death, the Quandes, members of their bridge club, had ended up with Dad's remains. Stan Quande had been on hand when Tom cleaned out the house and did the garage sale. Tom forgot to get the remains before he left for Alaska, which were in a closet, so Stan took them. We had quite a laugh about this, because Dad had always been so social. It seemed only reasonable that he'd still be visiting the neighbors! Anyway, John arranged to have The Doctor Agnes, K.E., buried with Dad's remains next to her.

While John began arranging things in Seattle, Ralph had to get The Doctor there. We had talked about having the mortician in Battle Ground drive her body to Seattle for the autopsy. However, they were swamped, and time was of the essence. So Ralph got the necessary permits and records, put The Doctor in the back of the van, and drove her to Seattle himself. The girls and I had quite a laugh over the thought of Ralph tooling down the highway, his country tunes on the radio, with Granny in the back of the van in a body bag!

Still in Battle Ground, I put together a collage of pictures of The Doctor for the funeral. Pictures of her in Australia, Alaska, Norway. Pictures with her babies, with her parents, in her homes, at the beach. Pictures of friends, weddings, parties. Pictures of her dancing with Tom just a few months ago.

Tom came down from Alaska the day before the funeral. Ralph and I met him in Seattle, and we all stayed the night with Homer and Betty.

Agnes LEONARD

Agnes Leonard was born on August 7, 1916 to Norwegian immigrants John and Ella Anderson, homesteaders near Lemmon, South Dakota. Her home was a one-room sod house.

In 1935 Agnes graduated from Northern Normal School in Aberdeen, S.D. She taught eight grades in a one-room schoolhouse for six years. She then moved to Washington. She married Charles Leonard in November 1942. She held a variety of positions, including administrative assistant at the University of Oregon, office manager and secretary/ bookkeeper for Yarrington's Mortuary in Seattle. She also worked in a variety of businesses with her husband. She is survived by her four children, Mary Lou Stowell, of Tacoma, WA; Charlotte Akin, of Battle Ground, WA; John Leonard, of Hayden Lake, ID; and Tom Leonard, of Anchorage AK; her sister, Gudrun Layton, of El Paso, TX; as well as seven grandchildren and five great-grandchildren.

Once affectionately called the Doctor Agnes, K.E. (Knows Everything), by her children, she died of Alzheimer's Disease on November 6, 1995 in Vancouver, WA.

Services will be held in Burien at St. Paul's of Shorewood Lutheran Church, 11620 21st S.W., on Thursday, November 9 at 1 P.M. Interment will immediately follow at Riverton Crest. Arrangements by Yarrington's Funeral Home. Memorials may be sent to The Development Office, Box 358220, The University of Washington School of Medicine, Seattle, WA 98195. Please designate gifts for Alzheimer's Research.—*Seattle Times,* November 8, 1995

The funeral was just as The Doctor would have wanted. My cousin Fatty came with her daughter. Mother's cousin, Magnihild, who had grown up on the neighboring farm and had once shared a doll with her, was unable to come. But Magnihild sent her son, Drew. Friends came from the neighborhoods she had lived in, the churches she had joined, from the bridge clubs. Mrs. Yarrington, wife of The Doctor's former boss, was there. Ann and Ken came, as did Janice and Joshua. Ana stayed at the foster care home for the day. All four of The Doctor's children attended, including some of her grandchildren and great grandchildren. Yarrington's did the arrangements. It was held in her church of many years, St. Paul's of Shorewood Lutheran Church. A vocalist, the pastor's wife, sang "In the Garden." Homer and Betty led those attending to share fond memories. The pastor led the liturgy, and the congregational hymn at the end, "The Old Rugged Cross."

Ralph gave a wonderful sermon. He read the story of Lazarus from scripture and then pointed out three things from the story as they related to The Doctor. First, Lazarus means "helpless." But God does not leave His people helpless. Angels escorted Lazarus to Heaven. Likewise, Mother was helpless. She had three angels who attended her, Ann, Ana, and Janice. Finally, there was the relationship between the Father and Lazarus. And this was what made the difference for him—he knew the Father, unlike the rich man in torment who did not. The most beautiful part of Ralph's sermon was when he showed how The Doctor had, to the end, greeted people with her arms out, child-like and a smile upon her face. It was a picture of her soul.

After the burial, we all went back to the church where the ladies there had prepared a light lunch of finger sandwiches, fruit, and beverages. It was truly just as The Doctor would have wanted it to be, and she was an expert when it came to funerals.

I was numb for some time after. By the time the funeral was over and I was back to work, it was nearly time for Thanksgiving. Ralph's sister, Marilyn, did Thanksgiving dinner. Then it was a blur trying to get ready for Christmas.

Ralph attended a hearing sponsored by the state regarding regulations on foster care homes. Nursing home lobbies, both wealthy and well-established, have quite an interest in regulating foster care. There's a lot of money and future potential in this battle. It would be a shame to lose family care settings for those in need of primarily custodial (rather than skilled nursing) care. Ralph had a chance to speak and to say so.

Ken and Ann remained friends. We got together for dinner and a movie before the holidays got under way.

Heather and Marc and Janelle all came home for Christmas, a real tonic for me. I still stopped in at the foster care home from time to time, just to say hello. On Christmas Eve Day, out on some last-minute errands, I stopped in again. The kittens were gone now, but Mama Cat had taken up residence on Pearl's bed. Hilda wore the pink sweater. Iris and Naomi sat in the living room watching TV. Janice had the house all decorated for Christmas. It was still a pleasant place to visit.

We had a traditional Akin Christmas, caroling with our neighbors, and then church on Christmas Eve. Christmas Day was quieter, but with a big dinner.

I'd had a sense of victory since Mom had died. Part of it was knowing she was at peace in Heaven, and with Dad. Part of it was knowing I'd done the best I could do...and that it was good enough. Part of it was that I had survived. When I'd had mono the first year caring for The Doctor, I had quipped to my doctor that she'd probably outlive me. He stopped me cold and said, "That's not funny." Of course I'd read all the books. I knew that often Alzheimer's patients outlived their caregivers. Indeed, Dad had died. However, the man speaking to me was looking at a 44-year-old woman. And he was quite serious. So I honestly felt it was a victory to just survive. I also had a sense, as I eased back into my own life, that it was good. I knew, from many regular walks, my neighbors and their dogs. Christmas gave me the sense that my own family was still in one wonderful piece. Although I'll never love the politics, I had a job that I loved. I'd not only survived, but I'd survived for some life of my own that was very worthwhile.

I'd had friends who had lost their mothers. I'd seen depression and tears. A friend from my old school, Hearthwood, would get a little teary every time she had something she wanted to talk over with her mother, but could no longer do. But I didn't feel that. I'd never had that kind of relationship with The Doctor to begin with. Even if I had, the talking-things-over would have stopped years before Mom was gone. Furthermore, I was more relieved than depressed. I did feel exhaustion.

Many of The Doctor's friends had written sympathy cards and expressed what a wonderful friend The Doctor had always been to them. She was the one who was there for them when they needed help. She was a comforter and a counselor, she provided hands-on help when needed. Indeed Mary Lou and I were sometimes jealous of The Doctor's friends who benefitted from that side of her. So while I knew that Mom had been a fabulous friend to others, it wasn't part of my relationship with her, and I didn't feel that loss either.

Still, there was a void in my life. It took me a while to define it. There was a child who was happy to see me when I came. We'd put on her hat and coat. I'd take her by the hand, and out we'd go together. We would walk or go and buy an ice cream sundae. We might drive in the country and sing on the way. We'd stop in at a farm where she would innocently steal fruit. She was very busy and yakky; she loved pretty things, and she loved a joke. If there was music playing, she would dance to it. She was so loving, such good company.

I was glad to have known this child-like woman. And I missed her.

Epilogue

As part of the study at the University of Washington, we agreed to a full autopsy, honoring Mom's wishes to make a contribution. Except for a scrape on her arm that happened when I was trying to move her a few days before her death, The Doctor's autopsy revealed the good condition of her skin, nails, and mouth—a testimony to the quality care she had received. It revealed emaciation, too. She weighed just 76 pounds. This led to respiratory failure. The muscles needed to breathe simply slowed to a stop. There was a trace of pneumonia in one lung. The other lung was collapsed. The underlying cause of death was listed as Alzheimer's. The tell-tale tangles and plaques were there in her brain. There was no other serious pathology. No cold, no flu, no cancer, no bad heart, no sign of a stroke. We had, then, a clean and clear case of Alzheimer's, without other complicating factors.

By the time Alzheimer's Disease had claimed The Doctor Agnes, K.E., her children were in middle age—from 41 to 51 years old. Mary Lou had grandchildren. She was on kidney dialysis, waiting for a kidney. Her husband had started his own business, which was prospering. My children were grown. Janelle was in college; Heather was married with a professional career. John's family had built a summer place on Hood Canal, not far from Seattle, where they went to relax, go boating and fishing. Their main home was still in Idaho, where Natalie and Andrew were junior high age. In addition to his businesses, Tom had remained active in Alcoholics Anonymous, holding out his hand to others trying to do the slow crawl out of addiction, two steps forward, one step back. Tom's family had recently purchased some river-front property in Alaska—also for a summer fishing place. His daughter, Jessie, nine, had been born during the year-long diagnosis process for The Doctor. So The Doctor had been afflicted for over ten years with the disease, being in the second stage—as is common—when she was diagnosed.

As a group, the Leonard kids had grown up with alcoholism, bankruptcy, divorce proceedings, and serious illness. We bore the scars of that upbringing into adulthood. There were fractures on us and between us that all the king's horses and all the king's men would never put together again. We had come to accept that by middle age.

Individually, each of us had established stable, first-and-only-marriage families, undoubtedly due in part to the triumphantly enduring marriage model we had observed growing up.

While we weren't a perfect family, I came to understand that the nature of my mother's life never depended upon our perfection. It depended upon a commitment to quality care and enough civility between us to deliver it. She had taught us well. When Alzheimer's Disease forced us all down the long, hard road to goodbye, we took good care of The Doctor.

Appendix A
Sample Copies of Monthly Reports
Sent to the University of Washington

MONTHLY PROGRESS FORM

PATIENT _Agnes Leonard_

ADPR # 040 _0 70_

DATE _5- 3- 88_

> **Please send for month circled.**
> Year _1988_
>
> JAN   FEB   MAR   (APR)   MAY   JUNE
>
> JULY   AUG   SEPT   OCT   NOV   DEC

Please complete the items below by checking the most appropriate answer to the following questions. Answer to the best of your ability and return this form to the Research Nurse using the enclosed, postage paid envelope.

Thank you.

1. How would you rate the patient's condition since last correspondence:

   _✓_ a. No change - relatively good

   _____ b. No change - relatively poor

   _____ c. Slightly better

   _____ d. Slightly worse

   _____ e. Much worse

2. Has the patient been hospitalized since last correspondence?

   _✓_ No

   _____ Yes; Number of Days: _____

3. Is the patient now in a nursing home?

   _✓_ No

   _____ Yes; Is this a change? _____No _____ Yes

Comments: _Depressed and shortage of Energy_
Plays bridge + visits with no problem

MONTHLY PROGRESS FORM

PATIENT _Agnes Leonard_

ADPR # 040 _0 7 0_

DATE _____

| Please send for month circled. |
| Year _1988_ |
| JAN   FEB   MAR   APR   MAY   JUNE |
| (JULY) AUG   SEPT   OCT   NOV   DEC |

Please complete the items below by checking the most appropriate answer
to the following questions. Answer to the best of your ability and return
this form to the Research Nurse using the enclosed, postage paid envelope.
Thank you.

1. How would you rate the patient's condition since last correspondence:

   _____ a. No change - relatively good

   _____ b. No change - relatively poor

   _____ c. Slightly better

   __✓__ d. Slightly worse

   _____ e. Much worse

2. Has the patient been hospitalized since last correspondence?

   __✓__ No

   _____ Yes; Number of Days: _____

3. Is the patient now in a nursing home?

   __✓__ No

   _____ Yes; Is this a change? ____No ____Yes

Comments: _Her sister is dying of Cancer._
Agnes is short on energy & complains of
Nausea & Stomach ache. Could all be
caused by stress. Have Dr. app Monday
the 8th of August

MONTHLY PROGRESS FORM

PATIENT _Agnes Leonard_

ADPR # 040 _0 7 0_

DATE _____

| Please send for month circled. |
| Year _1988_ |
| JAN FEB MAR APR MAY JUNE |
| JULY AUG SEPT (OCT) NOV DEC |

Please complete the items below by checking the most appropriate answer to the following questions. Answer to the best of your ability and return this form to the Research Nurse using the enclosed, postage paid envelope.

Thank you.

1. How would you rate the patient's condition since last correspondence:

  ✓ a. No change - relatively good

_____ b. No change - relatively poor

_____ c. Slightly better

_____ d. Slightly worse

_____ e. Much worse

2. Has the patient been hospitalized since last correspondence?

  ✓ No

_____ Yes; Number of Days: _____

3. Is the patient now in a nursing home?

  ✓ No

_____ Yes; Is this a change? _____ No _____ Yes

Comments: _We have had no company for the last 3 weeks. She seems to be doing much better. We are going to Reno for a few days beginning the 6th. We will be able to see how she handles it before making plans for Jan + Feb in Las Vegas + Arizona._

MONTHLY PROGRESS FORM

PATIENT *Agnes Leonard*

ADPR # 040 *O 7 O*

DATE *11-30-88*

| Please send for month circled. |
| Year *1988* |
| JAN FEB MAR APR MAY JUNE |
| JULY AUG SEPT OCT (NOV) DEC Gemini |

Please complete the items below by checking the most appropriate answer to the following questions. Answer to the best of your ability and return this form to the Research Nurse using the enclosed, postage paid envelope.

Thank you.

1. How would you rate the patient's condition since last correspondence:

   _✓_ a. No change - relatively good

   _____ b. No change - relatively poor

   _____ c. Slightly better

   _____ d. Slightly worse

   _____ e. Much worse

2. Has the patient been hospitalized since last correspondence?

   _✓_ No

   _____ Yes; Number of Days: _____

3. Is the patient now in a nursing home?

   _✓_ No

   _____ Yes; Is this a change? ____No ____Yes

   Comments: _Oct. + Nov have been good month._
   after all the Company - Sept and the death
   of her sister. We can get along real
   good at her level now.

MONTHLY PROGRESS FORM

PATIENT _Agnes Leonard_

ADPR # 040 _670_

DATE _1-2-89_

| Please send for month circled. |
| Year _1988_ |
| JAN FEB MAR APR MAY JUNE |
| JULY AUG SEPT OCT NOV (DEC) |

Please complete the items below by checking the most appropriate answer to the following questions. Answer to the best of your ability and return this form to the Research Nurse using the enclosed, postage paid envelope.

Thank you.

1. How would you rate the patient's condition since last correspondence:

   ___✓___ a. No change - relatively good

   _____ b. No change - relatively poor

   _____ c. Slightly better

   _____ d. Slightly worse

   _____ e. Much worse

2. Has the patient been hospitalized since last correspondence?

   ___✓___ No

   _____ Yes; Number of Days: _____

3. Is the patient now in a nursing home?

   ___✓___ No

   _____ Yes; Is this a change? ____No ____Yes

Comments: _She has done quite well during the holidays with a lot of company. She has decided to proceed with the research program. She goes into York Harp on 1-3-89._

MONTHLY PROGRESS FORM

PATIENT _Agnes Leonard_

ADPR # 040 _0 7 0_

DATE _____

| Please send for month circled. |
| Year _1989_ |
| (JAN) FEB   MAR   APR   MAY   JUNE |
| JULY   AUG   SEPT   OCT   NOV   DEC |

Please complete the items below by checking the most appropriate answer
to the following questions. Answer to the best of your ability and return
this form to the Research Nurse using the enclosed, postage paid envelope.
Thank you.

1. How would you rate the patient's condition since last correspondence:

_✓_ a. No change - relatively good

_____ b. No change - relatively poor

_____ c. Slightly better

_____ d. Slightly worse

_____ e. Much worse

2. Has the patient been hospitalized since last correspondence?

_✓_ No

_____ Yes; Number of Days: _____

3. Is the patient now in a nursing home?

_✓_ No

_____ Yes; Is this a change? ____No ____Yes

Comments: _I developed a serious Heart Problem_
after Vince. This has caused her a little
more fear than normal

MONTHLY PROGRESS FORM

PATIENT _Agnes Leonard_

ADPR # 040 _070_

DATE _4-16-91_

Please send for the month circled:

year _1991_

JAN	FEB	MAR	(APR)	MAY	JUNE
JULY	AUG	SEPT	OCT	NOV	DEC

Please complete the items below by checking the most appropriate answer to the following questions. Answer to the best of your ability and return this form to the Research Nurse using the enclosed, postage-paid envelope. Thank you.

1. How would you rate the patient's condition since last correspondence?

_____ a. No change - relatively good

_____ b. No change - relatively poor

__✓__ c. Slightly better

_____ d. Slightly worse

_____ e. Much worse

2. Has the patient been hospitalized since last correspondence?

__✓__ No

_____ Yes; Number of days: _____

3. Is the patient now in a nursing home?

__✓__ No

_____ Yes; Is this a change? _____ No _____ Yes

Comments: _Still dress + feeds herself_
She is very disoriented most of the time
Still knows every one

MONTHLY PROGRESS FORM

PATIENT _Agnes Leonard_

ADPR # 040 _070_

DATE _5-23-91_

Please send for the month circled:
year _1991_

JAN	FEB	MAR	APR	(MAY)	JUNE
JULY	AUG	SEPT	OCT	NOV	DEC

Please complete the items below by checking the most appropriate answer to the following questions. Answer to the best of your ability and return this form to the Research Nurse using the enclosed, postage-paid envelope. Thank you.

1. How would you rate the patient's condition since last correspondence:

_____ a.   No change - relatively good

__✓____ b.   No change - relatively poor

_____ c.   Slightly better

_____ d.   Slightly worse

_____ e.   Much worse

2. Has the patient been hospitalized since last correspondence?

__✓___ No

_____ Yes; Number of days: _____

3. Is the patient now in a nursing home?

__✓___ No

_____ Yes; Is this a change? _____ No _____ Yes

Comments: _She is not dreaming or imagining things as bad therefore much easier to live with._

Appendix B
Psychometric Test
Administered by Zilpha Haycox

PSYCHOMETRIC EVALUATION REPORT

PATIENT NAME: Agnes Leonard
DATE OF BIRTH: 8.07.16
AGE AT TIME OF TESTING: 78 years
EDUCATIONAL LEVEL: 14 years
OCCUPATION: Retired bookkeeper
PSYCHOMETRICIAN: Zilpha Haycox
DATE OF EVALUATION: 8.12.94
DATE OF TEST INTERPRETATION: 8.18.94

TESTS ADMINISTERED:

1.   Mattis/Coblentz Dementia Rating Scale
2.   Boston Naming Test
3.   Mini-Mental State Exam

EXAMINATION REPORT:

BEHAVIORAL OBSERVATIONS DURING TEST ADMINISTRATION
(As reported by psychometrician)

Charlotte - As you noted, your mother was tested in her room at the foster home where she resides. She was seated in a geri-chair, was neatly dressed in a warmup suit and was well groomed. She had a broad smile and held her arms out for a hug. She maintained a pleasant manner and showed no signs of distress during my visit. Throughout the session, her speech was dysarthric with a jumbling of sounds and words. She often perseverated, using single words picked up from my questions or converstion to her. She gazed seemingly uncomprehending of my purpose during the session and picked at the edges of her table. Anything that was placed before her was picked up and rubbed or fondled, however, she was unable to use anything in a purposeful manner.

She could not complete any task on the Mattis/Coblentz Dementia Rating Scale, such as repeating groups of 2 to 4 numbers, nor responding to either single or double commands, such as "open your mouth", or "shut your eyes." Nor could she follow my examples to do these tasks. She could not repeat any items one can find or buy at a supermarket. She was unable to name any of 10 items pictured individually on sheets of paper.(Boston Naming Test). On the Mini-Mental State Exam, she was able to follow a command to take a piece of paper from me with her right hand and fold it in half. This gave her a score of 2 out of a possible 30 points.

2.

Her disposition was sweet and she appeared at ease in the foster home owned and run by Annabell Rhodes. Her interactions with the owner were warm and completely stress free. The home was spotlessly clean, without any offensive odors or the smell of disinfectants. There was a relaxed air one gets in a loving environment and your mother appears to thrive in this wonderful atmosphere.

Charlotte, I was so impressed with your gentle, positive and loving attitude and acceptance of your mother. She just blossoms in your presence and that image will be with me for a long time. I am honored to make your acquaintance and loved our long discussion over lunch, which you so generously bought me. Please feel free to call me if you need any more information and we must continue our conversation! I look forward to reading your first draft of the book on you and your mother's experiences with Alzheimer's .disease.

Eric Larson's title: Eric B. Larson, M.D., M.P.H., Professor of Medicine

Sincerely,

Zilpha

Zilpha L. Haycox

A score of 144 is possible if someone is not impaired and attains a perfect score

Subject *Leonard*
Date *8.12.94*
Session _____

DEMENTIA RATING SCALE[1]

I. Attention:

A. Digit Span — (Maximum Forward + Backward = 8)
Forward: "I'm going to say some numbers and when I'm through, I want you to repeat the numbers in the same order .... Say them just the way I did .... Say what I say:

   2, 5   3, 1, 6   4, 7, 9, 2   Digits Forward ___2___

Backward: "Now when I say some numbers, I want you to say them backward ... For example, if I say 1,2, you would say 2,1. Understand? ... Ready?":

   1, 4   5, 3, 9   8, 5, 9, 3   Digits Backward ___0___
                                                      Score: ___0___ /8

B. Responses to Two Successive Commands: "I'm going to give you some commands ...
   Do what I say and then relax." *opened mouth repeatedly*
   1.   Please open your mouth and ~~close your eyes~~.
        Show me your tongue and raise your hand.
        (1 point each, max. score = 2; if patient can perform both double commands, skip
        C & D, giving max. credit)   Score: ___0___ /2

C. Responses to Single Verbal Commands: "I'm going to give you some commands. Do
   what I say and then relax."

   1.   Open mouth
   2.   Stick out tongue
   3.   Close your eyes
   4.   Raise your right hand   Score: ___0___ /4

D. Imitates: "Watch me ... Do what I do ... Imitate what I'm doing ... Do this."

   1.   Open mouth
   2.   Turn your head
   3.   Close your eyes
   4.   Raise your hand   Score: ___0___ /4

II. Initiation and Perseveration:

A. Verbal

   1.   "I'd like you to name all the things you can find or buy in a supermarket ... You
        have 1 minute to name as many different items as fast as you can."
        (Score # of items named in one minute -- max. 20. If 14 or more items are named,
        skip 2, 3, and 4, giving max. credit) ·

   (Continued on next page)

---

[1]   Coblentz, Mattis, Zingesser, Kasoff, Wisniewski and Katzman. <u>Archives of
      Neurology</u>, 1973, <u>29</u>, 299-308.

II. A. 1.   *gibberish*

1_____   6_____   11_____   16___0___
2_____   7_____   12_____   17_____
3_____   8_____   13_____   18_____
4_____   9_____   14_____   19_____
5_____   10_____   15_____   20_____ Score: ___0__/20

2.   "Look at me ... Look at what I'm wearing and holding. I'd like you to name all the
     things you see ... Name all the things I'm wearing or holding."

     (Score # of items named in one minute. Max. score = 8)

1_____   4_____   7_____   10_____
2_____   5_____   8_____   11_____
3_____   6_____   9_____   12_____   Score: ___0__/8

                                                   gibberish
3.   "Say 'bee' ... say 'key' ... say 'gee'. Now say 'bee, key, gee' 4 times.
     (Score 1 point for 4 consecutive repetitions. Max. score = 1)   Score: ___0__/1

4.   "Say 'bee' ... say 'ba' ... say 'bo'. Now say "bee, ba, bo' 4 times.
     (Score 1 point if patient can repeat series 4 times even with
     prompting. Max. = 1)   Score: ___0__/1

B. Motor

1. Double Alternating Movements

   a) Demonstrate: Left palm up, right palm down, then switch hand positions
      simultaneously several times.
      (Score 1 point for correct hand placement in 5 consecutive alternations. Max.
      score = 1 point)

      Time to do 5 consecutive alternations: ___*unable to follow command*___ Score: ___0__/1

   b) Demonstrate: Right hand clenched with palm down, left hand fingers extended
      with palm down. Switch hand positions simultaneously several times.
      (Score 1 point for correct hand placements in 5 consecutive alternations.)

      Time to do 5 consecutive alternations: _____|'_____ Score: ___0__/1

   c) Alternating tapping (demonstrate using the index finger of each hand): "Tap left,
      then right, then left like this." (Score 1 point for 10 consecutive alternations. Max. =
      1)

      Time to do 10 consecutive alternations: _____|'|_____ Score: ___0__/1

DRS Page 3

II. B. 2.   Graphomotor (If patient can do 2a, skip 2b, 2c and 2d, giving maximum credit)
            (1 point each correctly done)

   a.   "Copy this entire design. Start right here" (Point to the left side of paper
         approximately one inch from top)   Score: ___0__ /1

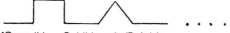
. . . .

   b.   "Copy this ... Put it here" (Point to paper approximately one inch below the
         ramparts reproduction)   Score: ___0__ /1

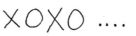

   c.   "Copy this ... Put it here" (Same -- one inch below)   Score: ___0__ /1

   d.   "Copy this ... Put it here" (Same -- one inch below)   Score: ___0__ /1

XOXO ....

III. Construction (If patient can do IIIA, give maximum credit, but complete all designs.)

   "Copy this. Put it here" (Point to patient's paper one inch from the top; indicate a one-inch
   spacing between the remainder of designs.)

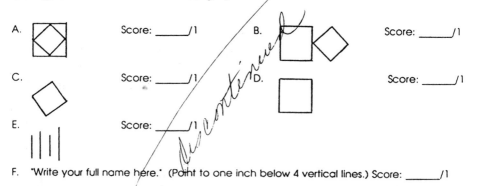

A.   Score: _____ /1   B.   Score: _____ /1

C.   Score: _____ /1   D.   Score: _____ /1

E.   Score: _____ /1

F.   "Write your full name here." (Point to one inch below 4 vertical lines.) Score: _____ /1

rest of test is not included

ID # 0 4 0   0 70

FOLLOW UP #: _____

DATE: 8.12.94

1 = CONTROL

2 = CO-PARTICIPANT

MAXIMUM SCORE	SCORE	
		ORIENTATION
5	(0)	What is the (year), (season), (month), (today's date), (day of the week)?
5	(0)	Where are we? (state), (county), (town), (hospital), (floor).
		REGISTRATION
3	(0)	Name three objects: 1 second to say each. Then ask the patient all 3 after you have said them. Give 1 point for each correct answer. Then repeat until all 3 are learned. Count trials and record.

TRIALS _____

ATTENTION AND CALCULATION

| 5 | (0) | Serial 7's. 1 point for each correct. Stop after 5 answers. (93, 86, 79, 72, 65)   WORLD (o) |

RECALL

| 3 | (0) | Ask for 3 objects repeated above. Give 1 point for each correct response. |

LANGUAGE

| 9 | (2) | Name a pencil and a watch (2 points) Repeat the following: "No ifs, ands, or buts". (1 point) |

Follow a three-stage command: Take a paper in your right hand, fold in half, and put it on the floor" (3 points)

Read and obey the following:

Close your eyes.

Write a sentence (1 point) *drew lines on folded sheet*
Copy design (1 point) *then continued to fold paper*

_02_ TOTAL SCORE

_02_ WORLD

#70

(Blessed Dementia Scale and Other Physical and Cognitive Changes)

A. Blessed Dementia Scale (ADL) (Information provided by informant)

1. Memory and performance of everyday activities:

On the left, rate subject's LOSS of ability to do the tasks listed below.
For each score of 0.5 or 1, indicate on the right whether reason is
physical (P), mental (M), or both (B).

Spoke E Annabell Rhodes

If unable to score, leave blank.

NONE	SOME	SEVERE	
0	0.5	①	A. perform household tasks
0	0.5	①	B. cope with small sums of money
0	0.5	①	C. remember a short list of items (e.g., shopping list)
0	0.5	①	D. find way about indoors (home or other familiar locations)
0	0.5	①	E. find way around familiar streets
0	0.5	①	F. grasp situations or explanations
0	0.5	①	G. recall recent events
0	0.5	①	H. Tendency to dwell in the past*

*(Score: 0 => none; 0.5 => sometimes; 1 => frequently)

2. Habits:

A. EATING

- 0 = Feeds self without assistance
- 1 = Feeds self with minor assistance
- ② = Feeds self with much assistance
- 3 = Has to be fed

B. DRESSING

- 0 = Unaided
- 1 = Occasionally misplaces buttons, etc., requires minor help
- 2 = Wrong sequences, forgets items, requires much assistance
- ③ = Unable to dress

C. TOILET

- 0 = Clean, cares for self at toilet
- 1 = Occasional incontinence, or needs to be reminded
- 2 = Frequent incontinence, or needs much assistance
- ③ = Little or no control*

3. TOTAL SCORE OF ALL BLESSED DEMENTIA SCALE ITEMS: [1 6 . 0]
(Maximum Score 17)

1/93

C2

References

Allen, J. Associated Press. (1998, November 19). Study offers clue to Alzheimer's. *The Columbian.* p. A3.

Alzheimer's disease. (1986). Report of the Secretary of Health and Human Services Task Force. Washington, DC.

Alzheimer's disease patient registry. (November, 7, 1994). [Letter]. Seattle, WA: Department of Medicine, University of Washington.

Armstrong, Mary. (1990). *Caregiving for your loved ones,* Elgin IL: David C. Cook.

Brownlee, S. (1991, August). Alzheimer's: Is there hope? *U.S. News and World Report,* pp. 40-6.

Cohen, D., and Eisdorfer, C. (1986). *The loss of self,* New York, NY: W.W. Norton.

Friend, T. (1995, June 28). Alzheimer's gene found. *USA Today,* p. 1.

Gruetzner, H. (1988). *Alzheimer's: A caregiver's guide and sourcebook,* New York, NY: John Wiley and Sons.

Hoffman, B. (1995). *Complaints of a dutiful daughter* [documentary]. "P.O.V." Public Broadcasting System.

Holman, J. (July, 1997). Can these pills help you live longer? *Readers' Digest,* p. 82.

Marmor, J. (1995, March). The age of dissonance. *Columns,* pp. 22-5.

Maugh II, T. *L.A. Times.* (1993, May 7). Report: Quick diagnosis of Alzheimer's possible. *The Columbian,* p. B7.

Nadler-Moodie, M. and Foltz Wilson, M. (July, 1998). Latest approaches in Alzheimer's care. *RN,* pp. 42-5.

Researchers find early sign of Alzheimer's. (1995, October 6). *The Columbian,* p. 2.

Silver, M. (1995, June 5). A light side of Alzheimer's? *U.S. News and World Report,* p. 68.

Ten warning signs. (July 6,1997). [Brochure]. Alzheimer's Association. [Online]. Available: http://www.alz.org.